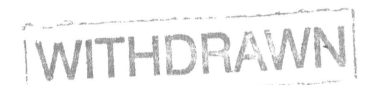

In place of the self: how drugs work

Ron Dunselman

translated by Plym Peters
and Tony Langham

HAWTHORN PRESS

In Place of the Self: How Drugs Work

Dutch edition *In plaats van ik*
© 1993 Uitgeverij Vrij Geestesleven, Zeist

English edition © 1995 Hawthorn Press
Published by Hawthorn Press
Hawthorn House, 1 Lansdown Lane, Lansdown,
Stroud GL5 1BJ, United Kingdom

Typeset in Plantin by Bookcraft, Stroud
Printed in the United Kingdom

Translated from the Dutch – *In plaats van ik: de verborgen werking van
drugs* – by Plym Peters and Tony Langham

Cover illustration
The Isenheimer Altar: The Temptation of St Anthony

Photo credits
p.38 FM Engel, Ansbach; pp.42–43 Musée Unterlinden,
Colmar (photo O. Zimmermann); p.116 Stern, ABC Press; p.203
Visions, ABC Press; p.83 ANP-foto; p.120 ANP-foto;
p.179 DPA/Pfund–ANP-foto;
p.199 Timothy Plowman.

British Library Cataloguing in Publication Data applied for

ISBN 1 869890 72 8

Contents

Foreword

It is difficult to define the world of drugs and drug users. This is true despite the fact that human beings have had so much experience of these substances, which apparently enable them to transcend themselves.

Nowadays, thoughts about the use of drugs are often determined by stereotyped ideas. The use of drugs is often associated with junkies, people who no longer belong, the drop-outs of society. This stereotyped perspective prevents us from seeing what is really happening in the world of drug users. In fact, the use of drugs is much more than a peripheral phenomenon of our modern society. For example, it also covers the use of alcohol, a substance which is very familiar to us in the west, and the increasing use of certain products from the pharmaceutical industry.

There is probably no other subject related to public health which attracts so much political interest, and sometimes also political conflict, as the use of drugs. There are a large number of regulations which aim, as far as possible, to restrict the availability of drugs. There is virtually no other field in which international co-operation exists on such a large scale as that of the use of drugs. International conventions, which have been drawn up following great efforts, serve as mandatory guidelines for governments throughout the world. The investments made to maintain and extend these conventions are constantly increasing. Unfortunately it seems that, despite all these efforts, the solution to the problem is receding. In increasing numbers of countries, the illegal use of drugs is a threat to the social order and to public health, particularly now that the use of drugs has also become an important contributory factor in the spread of the AIDS virus.

For the time being it does not appear as though worldwide policies and political ideas are able to cope with the illegal use of drugs. There is a danger that, if the current trends continue, this illegal use of drugs will become even further entrenched in our society. The technology for producing substances which influence consciousness is still developing and is increasingly accessible to many people. At the same time more and more people are affected by the economic factors which promote the use of drugs.

If we do not simply wish to accept this, it is important to start thinking differently about the use of drugs and about drugs themselves. This book opens a perspective on another way of thinking.

The book provides an insight below the surface into the everyday reasons for using drugs. It is a different sort of study into the nature and history of the substances which are used and the possible connections with the spiritual world.

For some readers this perspective may seem far removed from everyday reality; for many others, it will, I hope, serve as an invitation to reconsider.

Cees Goos
European Co-ordinator for Alcohol, Drugs and Tobacco,
World Health Organization

Editor's foreword

This is the first edition of Ron Dunselman's book *In plaats van ik* to be published in English. The statistics which appear in the main text relate, in most cases, to the Netherlands. Equivalent statistics, relating to the UK and to the USA, appear in the Appendix at the back of the book*. There are, however, several instances where equivalent statistics could not be traced. As Hawthorn Press wishes to produce a second English edition of this work, any relevant and appropriate data that readers can supply, relating to the English-speaking world, will be greatly appreciated.

Throughout the book, the drug user is referred to as either "he" or "she" in each alternate chapter, starting with "he" in Chapter 1.

* Footnotes indicated by a numeral refer the reader to the References; those indicated by a letter apply to the Appendix.

1

Introduction

In our century there has been an enormous increase in the consumption of alcohol and drugs. The Dutch Ministry of Public Health's memorandum on the problem of addiction (June, 1992) contained the following statement with regard to alcohol:

"In a quantitative respect, alcohol addiction is the most marked. Several hundred thousand Dutch people have serious problems controlling their consumption of alcohol, often resulting in serious physical and psychological problems."[1]

In addition, there are approximately 24,000 people addicted to hard drugs in the Netherlands,[2,a] while an estimated 500,000 people regularly use marijuana/hash (cannabis).[3,b] In fact, a growing number of people are having problems with the use of this drug.[4]

In 1987, approximately 250,000 people took daily sleeping pills or tranquillizers,[5,c] and in 1985 over 16,000 people died in the Netherlands as the result of smoking tobacco.[6,d] The number of people in Europe currently dying prematurely as a result of nicotine consumption is estimated to be between 750,000 and 1,000,000 per year.[7]

In addition, there is also a worldwide increase in the number of people who use cocaine and crack; for example, in North America the estimated figure is now 22 million people.[8,e] There are also the new synthetic drugs (designer drugs) which are attracting increasing attention; in the Netherlands an estimated 10,000 people are now regularly using Ecstasy (XTC).[9,f]

Reflecting on these figures, we come to the conclusion that there is a real drugs and addiction epidemic.

The prognosis is grim: if this development continues, by the year 2100, the number of drug addicts – i.e. people addicted to alcohol and other substances which change consciousness – in the industrialized world will exceed the number of people not addicted to drugs.[10]

What is this addiction, and what is the attraction of drugs which induces so many people to seek refuge in them? In other words, what are drugs?

What are drugs?

Basically, drugs are substances or compounds which lead to a change of consciousness. This change can take many different forms: drinking a beer to set your worries aside for a while, smoking a joint of marijuana/hashish to feel more relaxed, swallowing a tablet of ecstasy to be more open, active and communicative, shooting up heroin in order to dispel feelings of fear and sorrow. The characteristic aspect is always that the desired changes of consciousness are not brought about by our own inner activity, but are induced from outside by the effect of the substances taken.

Users do not change their consciousnesses themselves – they let the drugs do it for them. The change of consciousness is the aim; it is not a coincidental effect of taking the drug.

To summarize, it can be argued that drugs are substances or compounds which are deliberately used because they bring about a change of consciousness.

What is addiction?

Many people start the day by smoking a cigarette with their daily newspaper, wonderful! In the course of the day they have some nice cups of coffee, cigarettes to relax, a drink before dinner, a beer or a glass of wine with the meal, and a few pleasant hours in front of the TV, possibly finishing off with a sleeping pill before going to bed. That's okay, isn't it?

Looking at this example, it is clear that these pleasures can be distinguished from the everyday activities which we must carry out all our lives to keep our bodies healthy, such as breathing and sleeping. Breathing and sleeping are conditions of our existence and development on earth which are ordained by nature. If we do not carry out these activities, we neglect our bodies and eventually die.

And yet we are not addicted to these activities. For example, it would be ridiculous to say that we are addicted to breathing. We have to breathe, whether we like it or not. But we are not addicted to it.

The cups of coffee, cigarettes, the drink before the meal, the beer and the glass of wine are very nice of course, but basically we don't need them. Quite the reverse. The first time we smoke a cigarette or drink a glass of alcohol, the body protests violently, making us feel really sick. So the body's first healthy reaction indicates that the toxins are damaging to it rather than helpful to it. The fact that many of us go on to use them anyway is because repeated use proved to produce pleasant experiences and not because they were good for physical health and strength. They are used for pleasure, and not to sustain us.

Moreover, repeated use shows that the body gets used to these substances and that, as a result, increasingly high dosages are needed to produce the same effect (up to a certain toxic, i.e. lethal, level). This is called *tolerance*. For example, if at first one glass of wine was enough to produce a slight intoxication, after six months it may take four glasses.

The development of tolerance is accompanied by the development of *withdrawal effects*, which inevitably start to affect us painfully when we suddenly stop using the substance. For example, once a tolerance has been built up to alcohol, these withdrawal effects may consist of sweating, restlessness, irritability, trembling, insomnia, vomiting, muscular spasms, states of anxiety and depression, confusion and possibly even fits and hallucinations.

This is the situation in which the body has become dependent on the substance and can no longer function normally without it. This condition is known as *habituation*, which means there is a *physical* dependence revealed by two factors: tolerance and withdrawal effects.[11]

What was described above concerning the creation of a physical dependence also applies in broad terms for the development of a *psychological* dependence.

Obviously the morning newspaper and a few hours of watching the TV before going to sleep (but also, for example, sex telephone lines, stock exchange reports, pornographic magazines, working hard, and so on) are also not really necessary for our health, though we can give into them because they make us feel so good. As in the case of a physical dependence, the pleasure that is gained from these experiences can lead to an attempt to repeat the enjoyment.

However, when we realise after a time that we desire these pleasurable experiences so intensely that we do all we can to repeat them, this means that there is now also a *psychological* dependence on these activities which partly results from fear of the emptiness, dissatisfaction and restlessness caused by not satisfying the need.

A desire has developed in the soul. When we are no longer a match for this desire and can no longer resist it – when the desire has become stronger than our own individual strength, the strength of the Self to say no, then we are "hooked" and have become *addicted*.[12]

To summarize, we might say that we cannot become addicted to the nourishing food which we eat because it is necessary and, in the right quantities, it keeps our bodies healthy. The more we enjoy it, the better, because this means that we experience the beneficial effects even more effectively. In this respect we are like a king ruling over the realm entrusted to us (our body), as well as we can.

However, the roles are completely reversed when we take substances which we want only because of the pleasant sensations which they produce. (In fact, these pleasant sensations can be described in very broad terms; for example, it could be a pleasant sensation to stop experiencing an unpleasant sensation, such as inner emptiness, restlessness, anxiety, sorrow and withdrawal effects.)

If we constantly seek to reproduce these experiences, the desire in our soul – with the body in the background in the case of physical dependence – can eventually become an intolerant and insatiable tyrant which whines and rages if it doesn't get what it wants, when it wants. If we are unable to resist this, if we are unable to say no because the strength of our Self is not sufficient, it means we are dominated by our desire and have lost the freedom and independence of the king and have become slaves: we have become enslaved or addicted.

Thus addiction is a psychological dependence caused by an irresistible desire. This desire has a tendency to become increasingly dominant, so that in the end we think only about the substance involved, and all our feelings are entirely determined by it. We want only the substance concerned and we are completely taken over by it. On this subject, J.H. van Epen wrote: "The alcoholic's life is focused on alcohol; the heroin addict is always thinking about shooting up. Someone who is not addicted can return to daily matters after using the substance of his choice, but the addict is constantly preoccupied with his addiction. Therefore addicts often give an impression of leading a reduced existence."[13]

In his novel, *Het vangen van der draak* (Chasing the Dragon), Arie Visser's protagonist says: "The life of a junkie is dominated by desire and fulfilment ... The 'craving' (hankering, yearning) is the obsession of his existence, and is so strong that it dominates everything ... The tyranny of desire is so absolute that all other feelings pale in comparison, just as you cannot see the stars when the sun shines. It is only under the poppy's nocturnal canopy that normal feelings become conscious again ... How can you live like that? How can you be such a slave, day and night in the factory, on the conveyor belt of your desire for fulfilment?"[14]

What is drug addiction?

After a while an inner change takes place in a person who is addicted to drugs. At first, it was merely a matter of experiencing the satisfaction, the euphoria of an altered state of consciousness. But once he is addicted, the addict seeks drugs primarily in order to escape the feelings of torment which result from no longer being under the influence. The long-term addict does not take drugs to feel wonderful or "high", but rather to escape the misery of periods without drugs. Eventually the feelings of euphoria become weaker and weaker. The normal everyday consciousness of the long-term addict then consists of a drugged state and what seems a normal everyday state of consciousness, for someone who is not addicted, is torture for an addict.

An opium addict described this as follows: "The first time is a dream, an unbelievable experience of paradise, an encounter with the gods. The first few times are beautiful, so that you are reconciled with your existence. You are able to forgive, and at last you can breathe deeply and freely again. Then comes the time when you hardly notice when you take something, so you take more, and for a few days everything seems alright. However, it's not long until the day comes when a triple dose no longer has any effect. Even if you shoot up twice in quick succession, there's hardly any effect. Everything is reversed. It's only when you don't take anything that you notice anything – all the pain and the misery there is in the world. From that moment you pay a high price to feel normal. You suffer merely to avoid suffering. You run from one place to another, stealing, hustling, buying, chased by the police, and constantly ripped off by dealers. You buy dope, stick the needle in your arm ... and feel almost normal for a while, but then you have to score again, and so it goes on and on."[15]

2

Historical outline of drug use

We can now ask ourselves why drugs are used, considering the risks which they entail. In order to find an answer to this question, we must look to the past, because humans have tried to find ways of artificially changing consciousness since time immemorial. Drugs are actually as old as time. But why were they used in the past? To find the answer, this book adopts a spiritual perspective on the development of mankind.[1]

We have found four reasons for the use of drugs.

Back to the gods

In the first place, drugs were used to gain access to the world of the gods, i.e. to the world of extra-sensory creatures and experiences. In earlier times the reality of this extra-sensory world was just as obvious to ordinary consciousness as the external visual world is to our consciousness nowadays. We come across this in the Bible, the Bhagavad Gita, and many other religious texts whenever we read about the interaction between the gods and humankind in those times. There was not yet a clear distinction between the world of the gods and the world of humans, while the initiated priests, who felt at home in both worlds, organized life on earth in accordance with the will of the gods.

However, the world evolved, and gradually "twilight" fell on the world of the gods in human consciousness (Götterdämmerung), so that the original, self-evident orientation towards the divine and spiritual world was lost. Humans became more and more conscious of themselves, woke up to the earth, and learnt increasingly to become responsible for their own actions.

In order to restore the link with the divine, spiritual world, over the course of time, people were carefully prepared in many places throughout the world to achieve a state of consciousness which enabled them to make contact with the spiritual world once again. Drugs were used to facilitate this process. When the user had reached a spiritual state of consciousness by using drugs, as well as through other means, it was hoped that he could serve as a means to find out what was happening in the spiritual world, and what the gods intended.

Yet, for the users of the drugs themselves there were great dangers inherent in this method of seeking contact with the spiritual world. When they suddenly found themselves in a completely different state of consciousness, partly as a result of the drugs, they could become confused and overcome by fear. That is why the use of drugs was permitted only for people who had prepared themselves to tolerate the consequences of using drugs by means of lengthy and strict spiritual training, such as the initiated, those wanting to be initiated, oracle mediums, priests, shamans, medicine men and so on.

However, in the course of time, the "twilight" became darker and darker. The world of the gods fell increasingly silent, and humans, driven by their desires, became increasingly reckless in their use of drugs. For example, while the priest had entered a trance-like state of consciousness through drugs, the question is whether, after many centuries, the shreds of information which came to him from the spiritual world can still be considered to be reliable. These so-called "messages" from the gods were increasingly distorted, confused and ambivalent, so that it became extremely risky to consult the oracles and mysteries obtained in this way, or to take them seriously. The practice fell into disuse. In addition, the strict requirements of selection and preparation of those who used the drugs were weakened, with the result that larger and larger groups of people started to use drugs for pleasure during the rituals, ceremonies and feasts in order to blot out normal everyday consciousness and achieve a state of abandonment and ecstasy. In this way they had the extrasensory experiences without any preparation. Thus, from being sacraments used to enter the spiritual world after a long period of preparation and purification, drugs started to be taken purely for pleasure or "kicks", so that it was possible to have all sorts of unexpected and spectacular experiences while being completely unprepared and impure.

Nowadays, traces of this development can still be seen in the form of the so-called hallucinogenic drugs such as LSD, mescaline, other drugs which induce "trips", and, to a lesser extent, marijuana/hashish which take the user outside herself on a "trip" to an extrasensory world. The spirit of the past still prevails with regard to these drugs, as we read in the works of the great LSD prophet of the 1960s, Timothy Leary: "Three groups are bringing out the great evolution of the new age, which we are experiencing now. These are dope dealers, rock musicians and underground artists." Leary continues: "Of these three heroic mythical groups I believe that the dealers are the most essential and important. In years to come, television and film will show the 1960s dope dealer as an important figure. He will be the Robin Hood, spiritual guerilla, mysterious agent, who will take the place of the cowboy hero or the hero in police dramas. There is nothing new about this. Throughout the history of mankind, the shadowy figure of the alchemist, the shaman, the herbalist, the smiling wise man, who has the key to 'turn you on' and make you feel good, has always been the centre of religious aesthetic and revolutionary impulses. I think that it is the most elevated of all human professions, and I would strongly urge any creative young person who is truly interested in his own evolution and who wishes to help society to develop, to consider this old and honourable profession. The paradox of the just dealer is that he is selling you a heavenly dream. He is completely different from any other sort of trader because the goods which he is selling are freedom and joy. You expect your car dealer to drive a good car and your tailor to be well-dressed, and therefore it is self-evident that you expect a just dope dealer to radiate exactly the same joy and freedom which you are looking for in his products. Therefore the challenge for the dealer is not only that his product is pure and spiritual, but that he himself reflects the human light which he represents. Therefore you must never buy dope, never purchase the sacraments from someone who does not have the qualities which you are seeking yourself."[2]

However, the last few years have shown that all this was an illusion. The Robin Hood figure of the honourable dope dealer proved to be a criminal Mafia boss, who did not give freedom, but made slaves, and who, for a short period of joy, sold you subsequent depression and possible psychological disintegration. However, this does not mean that hallucinogenic drugs are not used anymore. On the contrary, in our time, when God is "dead" for many people, these substances have become very popular eye-openers to an extrasensory world. They answer a need for spiritual experiences, but they do this by recalling the tatters of a lost consciousness.

Towards the earth

From a historical perspective another reason for the use of drugs is in complete contrast to the reason given above: drugs were introduced because they actually give a first impetus to the above-mentioned distinction between the world of the gods and the world of humans. This applies particularly to alcohol.

Alcohol has been used for a long time in the evolution of humankind, as shown in two passages in the Bible: Genesis 9:20–21:

"And Noah began to be an husbandman, and he planted the vineyard:/And he drank of the wine, and was drunken; and he was uncovered within his tent."

Genesis 14:18:

"And Melchizedek, king of Salem, brought forth bread and wine: and he was the priest of the most high God."

Clay tablets dating from 6000 BC were found in the Nile delta, with recipes for the preparation of alcoholic drinks.[3]

Alcohol (wine) was the substance used particularly from the Egyptian/Babylonian civilization (approximately 3000 BC), and later increasingly during the time of the Greek civilization (from approximately 700 BC) to alter people's consciousness in such a way that the link with the gods was broken. By means of alcohol, people were driven towards their future state of consciousness, in which the gods made way for earthly realities and facts, in which people no longer "dreamed" in a mythical way, but thought in a rational way, and in which group consciousness would be replaced by a far more individual consciousness of the self. This new "earthly", everyday self-consciousness was stimulated – if necessary – by the sporadic and moreover, strictly regulated use of alcohol. It was known that long-term and unlimited use of alcohol entailed great dangers, and would eventually inevitably lead to an excessively earthly consciousness in which a person would forget their spiritual origins and would develop an inner hardness in their loneliness and selfishness. The first law on drinking alcohol was issued as early as 2225 BC by King Hammurabi (Babylon), in which he regulated and restricted the use of alcohol.

Later, the so-called cult of Dionysus developed in Greece and Asia Minor. This involved drinking wine at feasts, though again under strict conditions. At these celebrations the effect of the wine was experienced in company, and not individually, for this could result in alienation and melancholy. Balancing exercises were practised at these feasts, so that the participants could show that they were in control of their bodies, despite being under the influence. As a result of these efforts, they felt increasingly at home in their own bodies, in their "own piece of earth", which gave them a heightened sense of self-awareness. Another way of achieving this heightened sense of self-awareness was to drink so much wine that the physical consequences were experienced in the form of a terrible hangover. The hangover was what it was all about, i.e. the painfully heightened awareness of the participant's own body. For, in the cult of Dionysus, they were aware that the self-awareness produced in this way was necessary if people later wanted to take the path back to the spiritual world independently and from their own free will, retaining the self-awareness they had acquired. That is why the introduction of viniculture and the preparation of alcohol were based on the ancient mysteries. It was not so much for the benefit of the priests and the initiates themselves – as they had to acquire this new self-awareness through their own strength – but especially for many people in the local population who were pushed in this way to experience them-selves increasingly as individual and separate personalities.[4]

In the mysteries it was known that this process of severing oneself from the old ties should be a gradual one, if the effect was not to be destructive and shattering. The forced, unprepared and unregulated use of alcohol could inevitably lead to an excessively rapid break in the existing spiritual and social structures. This actually happened later on, particularly when alcohol was introduced to the Indians in the Americas and to many African nations. The effect was totally destructive as regards the social structures of these people, as de-scribed penetratingly by Albert Schweitzer, amongst others.

Thus gradually, in certain places dedicated to sacred mysteries, alcohol fulfilled a temporary "mission".

Until fairly recently (approximately 1800), with the exception of a few cases of excessive use,[5] alcohol in the western world retained this character of being regulated, (drinking at set times and during festive occasions), despite the disappearance of the sacred places. Subsequently the consumption of alcohol gradually got out of control and the concept of alcohol addiction first appeared.[6]

Finally, during our century, particularly after the Second World War, alcohol came to be used on a large scale and in a more permanent way. However, in the early 1980s there was a (slight) reversal of this trend in many countries.[7] The history of alcohol and the changing effect of this drug on human consciousness over the course of time are described in detail in chapter seven.

Stimulating effects

A third reason for the use of drugs has always been the increased level of performance, both physically (including sexually) and psychologically. By taking particular drugs the user is able to do much more than usual, and has greater physical as well as psychological powers at her disposal, so that she is able to break through her own natural limitations in this way. These drugs are known as stimulants.

I give the following example. According to an Inca sage, Marko Kapak, the son of the sun, gave the coca shrub to the people in the distant past (probably approximately 3000 BC) in order to cheer up those who were sad, to give new strength to the weary and exhausted, and to still the hunger of the hungry. In 1555, the conquistador Auguste Zárate wrote in astonishment to his king that by chewing the leaves of the coca plant, the Indians were able to "stay underground in the mines for 36 hours without sleeping and without eating."[8] In 1859, cocaine was first extracted from the leaves of the coca plant, and this stimulating drug, which produces a rush of energy, gained popularity in waves (first wave: after 1860; second wave: from the First World War up to the "Roaring Twenties"; third wave: particularly in the 1980s) to become an overwhelming stimulant.

Here is another example. In China, from the 6th century AD, large numbers of people enjoyed the mild stimulating effect produced by the leaves of the tea bush, which contained caffeine. Although the tea plant was probably known as early as 3000 BC, its stimulating effect was discovered only many centuries later, as illustrated by the following legend: "Bodhidarma, one of Buddha's pupils, was overcome by sleep during his nighttime meditation. Because he did not wish to be tormented by this human weakness again, he cut off his eyelids and threw them on the ground. They took root, and very quickly grew into a bush with green leaves. When with great astonishment Bodhidarma tasted the leaves the next morning, he was suddenly wide awake and no longer tired. He had discovered the power of tea."[9]

In Europe, caffeine appeared in the form of coffee. This mild, stimulating drug which keeps tiredness at bay, and encourages quick, clear and coherent thought, came from the Arab world. There are two legends about the origin of coffee. According to the first, there was once a herdsman guarding a herd of camels in Abyssinia, the land of origin of the coffee bush (Ethiopia). One night he noticed that the animals were more restless than they had ever been before. The next morning he discovered that the camels had completely stripped bare a number of bushes. He told the monks at the nearby monastery of Kaffa about the events of the night. They studied the bushes, and ever since they have used the leaves to make an infusion which kept them awake during their prayers and meditations.[10] According to another legend, the prophet Mohammed was able to drive out his tiredness with the coffee brought to him by the Archangel Gabriel.[11]

Initially the leaves of the coffee bush were used, but later (approximately 1000 AD) this changed, and the fruit was eaten (berries). Even later – in 1511, to be precise – the first coffee was prepared in the Islamic centres of Mecca and Medina, using the dried and ground seeds (beans). After this, the plant rapidly spread to Europe; the first coffee house opened in Constantinople (now Istanbul) in 1517. However, the new drug encountered a great deal of opposition; priests called it "the black drink of the devil which would bring hellish torture to man", and twenty-five years later the Grand Vizier of Constantinople had coffee drinkers sewn into leather bags and thrown into the sea.[12] The new drug was not legalized quickly! Coffee only really became popular in the course of the next few centuries when Turkish soldiers used strong coffee diluted with a dash of opium as a stimulant during their campaigns in Europe. This "heroic water" drove out fatigue, gave extra energy and strength (coffee), as well as dispelling feelings of fear (opium). However, the opposition continued to exist even against pure coffee. For example, in England a "women's petition" was issued in 1674, expressing indignation about the coffee houses, which did not admit women, where men spent their money on a drop of "mean, black, thick, dirty, bitter, stinking, disgusting, muddy water. It makes the men as infertile as the desert."[13] The petition actually asked for the drinking of coffee to be prohibited for anyone under the age of sixty!

However, when the Turks were defeated in Vienna in 1683, and the conquering Christians seized a booty of 10,000 bags of coffee, there was no stopping it, and despite all the regular prohibitions, prison sentences and so on, coffee eventually developed to become the most popular drink of the people in many countries.

Stimulants were always very popular in wartime. Enormous numbers of "combat pills" were taken both by the Nazis and by the Allies during the Second World War. These counteracted fatigue, gave courage and encouraged aggressive behaviour. For example, British and American soldiers swallowed more than 150 million amphetamine tablets.[14] After the war, large supplies of pep pills came on the Japanese market from the army dumps; the result was a wave of addiction of an estimated 500,000 to 1,000,000 users (in 1950). In 1954, 55,000 people were arrested, but after this, even strict laws were unable to put a complete stop to the use of these drugs.[15]

In the world of sport these drugs have also become popular for artificially increasing performance levels. This practice is known as "doping".

Drugs as medicine

In the fourth place, drugs have been used since time immemorial as medicines. In many cultures the shaman (magician) was also the medicine man who could use his drugs to induce religious ecstasy as well as for curing people. In their book, *Pflanzen der Götter, die magischen Kräfte der Rausch und Giftgewächse* (The Plants of the Gods, the Magical Powers of Intoxicating and Toxic Plants), Schultes and Hofmann write: "For example, in native medicine the hallucinogenic drugs which enable the native medicine man, and sometimes also a patient, to contact gods and demons, are also used as first class medicines. The role which they play is valued much more highly than that of medicines which have a direct effect on the body. Therefore for most native people they have gradually become a fixed starting point of 'medical treatment'."[16] One example of this is marijuana/hashish (cannabis), which has been popular with many African and Asian tribes for centuries, as a sort of universal medicine for all sorts of complaints and diseases. For example, 5000 years ago the Chinese emperor and herbalist, Shen Nung, recommended cannabis for treating malaria, beri-beri, constipation, rheumatic pains and women's complaints.[17] In India this "gift from the gods" was used, amongst other things, to stimulate the mind, prolong life, improve the critical faculties, bring down a fever, help people to sleep, and to combat dandruff, headaches, manic states, whooping cough, earache, venereal diseases and tuberculosis.[18]

In our time, drugs are also used as medicines: for example, the opiates, morphine and heroin, are excellent painkillers (anaesthetics), and LSD and other hallucinogenic drugs have been used from time to time to treat patients suffering from serious trauma, such as the so-called "concentration camp syndrome" (introduced by Professor Bastiaans in the Netherlands). In addition, there are the countless sleeping pills, valium-like tranquillizers and anti-depressants which help users to make their lives tolerable; as well as heroin to drive out fear, shame and sorrow, alcohol to banish anxiety, and speed and cocaine to combat inner passivity, emptiness and insecurity.

This brings us to one of the most important contemporary reasons for the use of drugs, viz. the use of drugs as self-medication in order to drive out undesired psychological conditions.

3

The use of drugs in our time

As we saw in the previous chapter, drugs have existed since time immemorial, though the phenomenon of drug addiction is much more recent.

With regard to alcohol, the concept of alcohol addiction first appeared in about 1800. Up until then, the most damaging result of the use of alcohol was drunkenness, which was considered to be immoral behaviour and a cause of many diseases. Later it came to be considered as a disease in its own right. However, during the nineteenth century the long-term use of alcohol increased dramatically. On the one hand, this was caused by the lack or poor quality of drinking water in the growing industrial centres; it was actually necessary for people to drink beer, wine and distilled drinks if they were not to fall ill. On the other hand, a large proportion of the population was exposed, at that time, to poor housing, working and living conditions. This encouraged alcohol consumption as a form of consolation to deal with the hardship and pressures of life. The graph on the following page shows the pattern of alcohol consumption in the Netherlands since 1880.

There has been a striking increase in consumption since the Second World War. The consumption of alcohol per head of population is now significantly higher than it was in the decades just before the turn of the century, which were themselves characterized by high consumption related to poor social conditions.

A more detailed study of Graph 1 reveals:
- the high level of consumption at the end of the last century;
- the marked decline since that time (because of an improvement in social conditions and large-scale campaigns to combat the use of alcohol);
- the enormous increase after the Second World War until the mid-1970s;

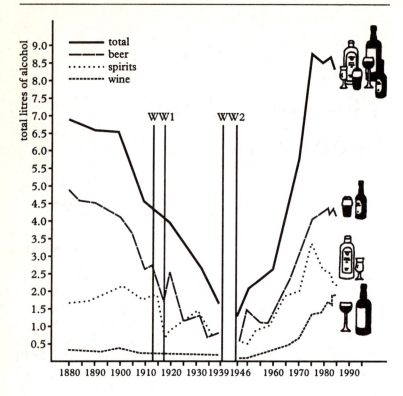

Graph 1:   Alcohol consumption in the Netherlands in litres per head of population, 1880–1985[1,a]

– the stabilization and slight reversal which occurred afterwards in
   the pattern as a whole.

An examination of the development – from the time when the
greatest increase started in 1960 – shows that the most marked
increase in alcohol consumption took place between the years 1966
and 1975 (see Graph 2 on the following page).

Another graph, showing the estimated number of excessive drinkers
in the period 1960–1990, also shows that the greatest increase in the
average amount of alcohol consumed daily took place between 1966
and 1975 (see Graph 3 on the following page).

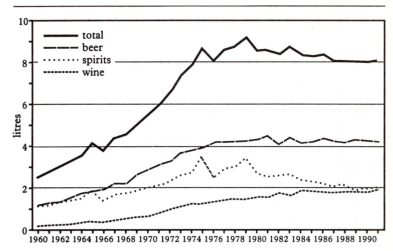

Graph 2 Alcohol consumption per head of the population in the Netherlands 1960–1991[2,b]

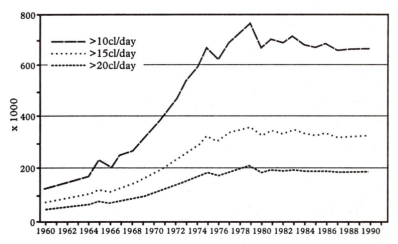

Graph 3 Estimated number of excessive drinkers in the Netherlands 1966–1990[3,c]

A study of another drug, viz. nicotine (tobacco), reveals a similar development: from the mid-1960s there was a marked increase in consumption, particularly between 1966 and 1979, followed by a decline, and in recent years another slight increase in cigarette smoking. There has been a stabilization and decrease in the use of pipe tobacco/rolling tobacco since 1983, after an initial increase (see Graph 4).[d]

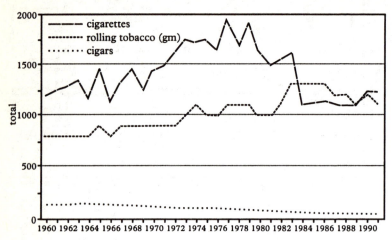

Graph 4   Tobacco consumption per head of the population of the Netherlands, 1960–1991[4,e]

For most other drugs there has also been a tremendous increase in consumption since the late 1960s, as shown in Table 1 on page 29.[5] There has also been a striking increase in the amount of cocaine seized. In 1988, more cocaine than heroin was seized for the first time. In addition, the seizing of hashish reached record heights in 1990.

To summarize, it may be stated that:

1. Since the mid-1960s there has been a tremendous increase in the use of drugs, including alcohol – though the increase in alcohol consumption started earlier – and particularly in the use of new drugs such as marijuana/ hashish, LSD, heroin, amphetamines and, later, cocaine.

2. Since the second half of the 1980s, the pattern has stabilized, followed by a slight reversal in the use of most drugs with the exception of cocaine, marijuana/hashish, and recently alcohol. Nevertheless, the use is still extremely widespread.

   Some estimates are given below.

a. In 1990, 664,000 Dutch people drank a minimum of eight glasses of alcohol per day; this included 326,000 people who drank at least 12 glasses of alcohol per day, of whom 186,000 people drank on average more than 16 glasses per day.[7]

Table 1   Main substances referred to in the Opium Act, seized in the Netherlands 1972–1991[6,f]

Year	Heroin kg	Cocaine kg	Hashish kg	Marijuana kg	Amph. kg	LSD doses
1972	2	–	2,000	315	–	7,800
1973	25	4	5,749	145	–	4,900
1974	28	7	5,312	194	–	12,200
1975	59	1	6,913	488	–	19,900
1976	171	2	9,888	246	43	52,000
1977	195	1	22,828	1,539	138	2,772
1978	87	4	12,204	526	50	7,900
1979	94	11	15,198	2,721	17	1,083
1980	116	46	14,200	1,410	11	4,686
1981	173	13	13,863	4,397	27	6,678
1982	226	37	11,536	3,031	129	48,128
1983	150	59	25,300	3,780	66	5,066
1984	144	180	18,845	10,759	39	10,531
1985	364	124	14,112	20,789	42	128,246
1986	542	274	35,296	12,559	86	3,618
1987	517	406	31,998	16,619	125	13,250
1988	510	517	46,221	22,017	53	468
1989	492	1,425	14,071	28,234	65	8,075
1990	532	4,288	90,000	19,752	47	5,146*
1991	406	2,488	73,962	22,330	128	1,630

* In addition to more than 5000 LSD trips, 54 grammes of LSD were seized, which is enough for 700,000–1,000,000 trips

b.   The number of people using hard drugs in the late 1980s, early 1990s in some European countries (see Table 2, page 30):
c.   Also see the figures shown in the introduction.[10]

The question arises as to why drugs have become so attractive to so many people in the last third of this century. What has changed in the human psyche for people to seek refuge in all sorts of substances as an external means of evoking particular experiences in the soul?

In order to find an answer to this question, we should turn to developments in the recent past. It is clear that since the 1960s there have been profound changes in our social and cultural life. Up to that time, the patterns of our thoughts, feelings and desires were determined to a far greater extent by gender, family, social class,

Table 2   Users of hard drugs in Europe in about 1990[8]

Countries	Estimated number of people using hard drugs	Population (in millions)
France	120,000–150,000	56
Italy	100,000–200,000	57
West Germany	60,000–80,000	61
Great Britain	60,000–80,000	56
Soviet Union	46,000*	280
Greece	40,000–50,000	10
Poland	38,000	37
Switzerland	28,000–56,000	7
The Netherlands	20,000*	15
Sweden	10,000–14,000	8
Yugoslavia	10,000*	23
Denmark	6,000–8,000	5
Norway	5,000	4

* Registered with the addiction support centres.

profession, religion or the community. However, in the course of the 1960s things increasingly changed. The late 1960s were a time of great upheaval in our culture; the time of the student revolts, first in Paris, and later also in other parts of the world. "L'imagination au pouvoir" (Power to the imagination) – things had to change. We wished to get things moving. We wanted to determine for ourselves where we were going, on the basis of our own ideas. Attempts were made to expand consciousness, and for many people, drugs (particularly LSD and marijuana/hashish) seemed to be the perfect solution for this. Traditions were queried, and many traditions learned by rote were turned inside out. Some obvious examples of this include the questioning of traditional role patterns; relationships with authority in the family, school, university and industry; the movement for the emancipation of women and suppressed minorities, the changes in sexual morality, with sexual relations becoming freer and more diverse, the decline in church attendance, and so on.

In this respect, traditions and customs have two characteristics which are important. On the one hand, they prevent the psyche from being free, and obstruct an inquiring attitude to reality. On the other hand, they provide the soul with an inner cohesion because they enable people's ideas, customs and motives to be interrelated. In other words, the tradition ensures that ideas and desires are interrelated and form a certain unity within the personality. (In this case you act on the basis of the idea that this is the way you ought to act.) When the formative strength of tradition disappears, this not only leads to freedom, but also to the need to create an inner relationship between ideas, feelings and desires, using one's own resources. Perhaps one of the characteristic qualities of people today is that we find that what we think or feel does not necessarily accord with what we want. Or what we feel conflicts with what we do, or we may find: "I think or do one thing, but in my heart I feel another."

Thinking, feeling and the will each start to live their own life; they start to become emancipated, as it were, and every day there is a new task to recreate the interrelationship between these three forces in the soul.

Up until the 1960s, culture and traditions were responsible for doing this to a much greater extent. But the break with traditions created a break in the soul which, on the one hand, gave us the freedom to create our own content, interrelationship and cohesion of thinking, feeling and the will. On the other hand, the question arose as to whether we had enough strength to do this on our own with the resource of our own Self.

However, drugs can also do this for us. Drugs can temporarily activate, strengthen or emphasize one or more of these three forces of the soul. Drugs can stimulate (associative) thinking, direct our feelings in a particular direction, or strengthen the will and our performance.

With regard to *thinking* and the visual imagination connected with it, the following drugs exist to stimulate it:
- Cocaine and amphetamines (speed) affect the user in his head; associations are made with lightning speed and the user feels extremely clear-headed.
- Alcohol also has this effect for a short time after the initial drink.
- Caffeine – and coffee in particular – stimulates rapid, clear and coherent thinking in a mild way.
- LSD, mescaline and other drugs used for tripping, and to a lesser extent, high doses of marijuana/hashish, produce altered perceptions and inner imagery; opium also does this, though in a far more dreamy way.

Recently we have seen the emergence of "smart" drugs, also known as "smarties" or "learning pills", which allegedly stimulate the functioning of the brain (including the hormonal compound vasopressin, and the substances, hydergine and piracetam). Most of these medicines were developed for older patients with degenerative brain functions but, despite the considerable side effects, they are increasingly taken by healthy young people, particularly scholars and students who wish to improve their learning performance.

With regard to *feeling*, the following drugs are available.

Marijuana/hashish produces much stronger feelings than those which are felt normally, varying from the more intense emotionally experienced perceptions and observations which can produce a happy mood, to the sweet dream or shadowy change of consciousness which gives a sense of being relaxed, and eventually often ends in sleep. That is why it is such a welcome solution to many young people whose souls feel shrivelled up as regards feeling, because only their thinking functions are being addressed and developed (particularly as a result of an education that is excessively one-sided and focused in the intellect). But those who wish to lose themselves in overactivity (a one-sided dominance of the will) may also experience a sense of well-being and tranquillity as a result of using marijuana/hashish.

Alcohol also produces strong feelings and, because it dispels inhibitions, it serves for many people as a drug to promote contact and stimulate conviviality. In P.H. Esser's words[11], it is a "social lubricant", and "strong drinks" also produce feelings of strength, self-confidence, over-confidence and aggression.

Cocaine and speed elevate moods and also produce a feeling of self-confidence and euphoria. They give a sense of superiority. Crack, which is made from cocaine, achieves this effect even more quickly and powerfully.

Sleeping pills and tranquillizers reduce anxiety and instill a feeling of indifference, calm and rest, while nicotine produces a mild sense of tranquillity when the smoker feels tense or nervous.

Opium, the opiates, morphine, heroin, and also the synthetic surrogate, methadone, dull the unpleasant sensations of fear, sorrow, pain, shame and so on, to a greater or lesser extent, and reduce consciousness to a relaxed feeling of indifference and physical well-being.

When morphine, heroin, cocaine or speed are injected into a vein (mainlined), this intense euphoric feeling or "flash" is produced within a few seconds.

With regard to *the will*, there are the following drugs: stimulants, such as amphetamines (speed, pep pills), artificially produce will-power and give the user a sense of increased energy.

Caffeine does this in a mild way, so that there is also a sense of physical stimulation.

Cocaine permits the body to perform at a higher physical level, as Freud described: "You notice that your self-control increases, and that you are full of vitality and the will to work. In other words, you are quite normal, and after a while you can hardly believe that you are under the influence of a narcotic drug. Lengthy and intense mental or physical labour can be carried out without a trace of fatigue." Freud sent his fiancée some cocaine and wrote to her in a letter: "Beware, my princess, when I come to you. I will kiss your cheeks until they are red, and make you eat until you are plump again. And if you are obstreperous, you will see who is strongest, a sweet little girl who does not eat enough, or a big rough man who has taken cocaine. During my last black depression I took some more coca, and a small dose helped me to get over it completely, quite miraculously. I am now busily collecting literature to write an ode to this magic drug."[12]

Finally, nicotine is a light stimulant, if the smoker is feeling slightly passive or listless.

Thus we see that drugs are able to temporarily place one or more of the three forces of the soul in the foreground. In this way, drugs can be a solution to the inner challenge involved in the emancipation of each of the three areas in the soul: thinking, feeling and the will. In the case of repeated use, this entails the risk that the core of our personality, the Self, is increasingly deactivated, and that the drugs – rather than the Self – start to determine the interrelationship and cohesion between thinking, feeling and the will. In this case the drugs solve the inner challenge for us, taking the place of the Self, which is put out of action to a greater or lesser extent. Because of this, the Self is less able to develop, and eventually it will increasingly lack the strength to achieve the interrelationship between thinking, feeling and the will, so that the temptation and need to do this with the help of drugs merely increases, ultimately resulting in drug addiction.

In extreme cases, this results in the contemporary long-term addict of hard drugs: the so-called "poly" drugs user, who is constantly concocting a meal of drugs to provide him with the required content, strength and interrelationship of the three areas of the soul. In doing so, he looks for the most ideal combinations, the best "cocktails". In his autobiographical novel, *Junkie*, William Burroughs describes this with regard to the simultaneous combination of feelings of tension and relaxation when he is preparing a "speedball":

"I held a match under the spoon until the morphine had dissolved. You never heat cocaine. I added a bit of cocaine on the point of a knife, and immediately saw the cocaine dissolve like snow when it comes into contact with water. I wound a frayed tie around my arm. I breathed more quickly with excitement, and my hands shook. 'Can you fix me, Ike?' Old Ike carefully felt along the vein with a finger, holding the syringe between the thumb and fingers. Ike was good. I hardly felt the needle slide into the vein. Dark red blood spurted into the syringe. 'O.K.', he said, 'let it go'. I loosened the tie and the syringe emptied into my vein. The cocaine hit my head, a pleasant dizziness and tension, while the morphine spread through my body in relaxed waves. 'Was it good?' Ike asked, smiling. I answered, 'If God made anything better, he kept it for himself.'"[13]

Various combinations are possible in a single drug which can regulate the forces of thinking, feeling and the will in a particular way.

A fairly recent example of this is ecstasy (XTC), also known as MDMA: (3.4 *m*ethylene *d*ioxy*m*ethyl *a*mphetamine), which came to the Netherlands in 1988. The drugs researcher, August de Loor, wrote about this drug:[14] "Ecstasy has a consciousness expanding effect. This should be seen as its main effect. It is this effect that concerns the consumer. The energy produced by ecstasy should be seen as a carrier. The carrier activates the main function, but there are other factors. Logically one would expect that if they are added together they would repel each other, for in fact they are opposites. The special quality of Ecstasy is that this does not happen. The opposing influences do not cancel each other out. In fact, they seem to enhance each other. The energy effect increases the main effects. As a result, the consumer does not experience any hallucinogenic effects. The consciousness-expanding side breaks down the energy aspects. Therefore the sense of being swung to and fro, the peaks and troughs of uncertainty which are characteristic of amphetamines, are not experienced with Ecstasy. The consumer feels only a slight feeling of energy, so that the effect of consciousness expansion is experienced more clearly."

He drew the diagram shown on the following page.

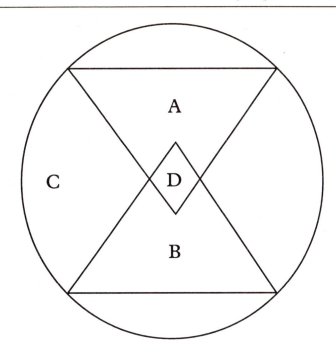

A is the consciousness expanding side of Ecstasy and should be seen as the main effect. (*Thinking*)

B is the energy aspect of Ecstasy and should be seen as the "carrier" of the main effect. (*The will*)

C ensures that A and B overlap; this overlap, *D*, is particular to Ecstasy. It diminishes the effect of A and B; D is also known as Ecstasy's safety valve.

Ecstasy *feels* good, because the initial phase is followed by a warm feeling, both physical and spiritual, that is described as a pleasant social feeling."[15] (*Feeling*)

To summarize, it is clear that Ecstasy is able to combine the areas of the soul – thinking, feeling and the will – in a unique way that is very pleasant for the user.

It is to be expected that in the future many other similar substances will become available, i.e. drugs which can manipulate the consumer's thoughts, feelings and will in the most subtle and distinct – and even powerful – ways. This reminds us of A. Sahini's vision of the future, which he describes at the beginning of his book, *Synthetische drugs* (Synthetic drugs).

"One day, in the still fairly distant future, cheap drugs will be available with which man can choose to regulate his feelings of pleasure and discontent, his periods of productivity and rest, without in any way harming either himself or society.

We already – at least approximately – have the required neuro-physiological and chemical knowledge and the chemical components to produce these future bringers of happiness and relaxation."[16]

However, each and every one of these new drugs will have in common the fact that, just like the present drugs, they will take the place of the Self to a greater or lesser extent – giving the Self a holiday, as it were. The drugs take over a number of the tasks and functions of the Self, and in this respect replace the Self.

This raises the question: "How can drugs do this?" In other words, what are the effects of the various consciousness changing substances on the human organism, and how do they work? How is this effect achieved?

The following chapters will deal with these questions in detail. The description of the effects of the various drugs will follow a description of the history of the drug concerned. This is the best way for us to know the drugs.

4

LSD

LSD is produced synthetically by adding a diethylamide group to lysergic acid, which is derived from ergot. This produces *Lysergic* acid *d*iethylamide, abbreviated to LSD,[1] which is extremely volatile in light and air. When taken orally, the strong effects start after approximately three-quarters of an hour; then it loses intensity to return with full intensity, and recede and return until this rhythmic pattern passes after eight to twelve hours.

Ergot

The basic raw material for LSD is a plant, ergot. What sort of plant is this? What does it look like? Ergot is a fungus which grows predominantly in the flowering of an ear of rye (see photograph on p.38), and to a lesser extent in the flowers of other cereals. It prevents the ear of rye from forming healthy fruit in the normal way (grains of rye), and in this respect it is therefore a parasitic fungus which weakens the host plant – the rye – and eventually makes it infertile for the benefit of its own reproduction. This reproduction takes place, inter alia, when the fungus dissolves in countless spores in the place where the rye flowers, so that it is hardly of a "material" nature.

This has the following implications. The inflorescence of a plant can be seen as the least material part of its physical manifestation, which is expressed both in the growth of the delicate, sometimes transparent, thin petals, and in the formation of the often microscopically small grains of pollen on the stamens. The plant virtually disappears in a material sense in these grains of pollen, as though it dissolves or "dematerializes". But it is precisely by means of these extremely small grains of pollen that it is able to "expand" enormously at the same time, because its *effect* can now stretch out over a large area of many square miles when the wind and insects disperse the pollen over large distances to the sticky stigmas of other flowers. In the grains of pollen the plant disappears almost completely in

---

Photograph overleaf: The mould (ergot), the natural raw material of LSD.

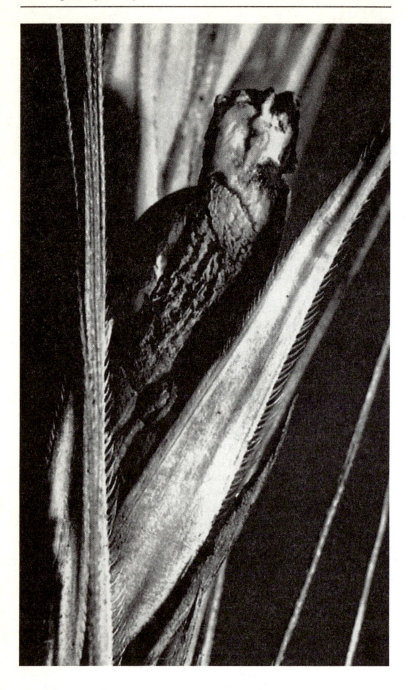

terms of size and its material quality, at the same time as being almost infinitely expanded through the effect of the pollen. It is as though it is diluted or "homeopathized" in space, in Goethe's words, assuming its most refined state.

Ergot is particularly attracted to this process of pollination, this movement of dematerialization and this solution of substance in space, which takes place in the flower of the ear of rye. Its spores are distributed on the stigmas of the waiting rye flowers, where they develop to become mycelium and eventually the extremely poisonous violet-black, banana-shaped grains of ergot, as well as reproducing themselves at the ends of the mycelium filaments by partially dissolving into countless new spores. The ergot lodges in the movement of the dematerialization and dissolving of the ear of rye. It feels very comfortable there, for the process of a substance dissolving is familiar to it, though this is as a parasite on the host plant, the rye, which it eventually weakens and deforms.

Ergot in history

The first historical mention of the plant ergot (*Claviceps purpurea*) was made in approximately 600 BC, when the Assyrians described it as a "harmful boil in the ear of corn".[2] The holy books of the Parsees (dating from approximately 350 BC) mention ergot: "Amongst the disastrous things created by Ariman, there is harmful grass which causes prolapse of the womb in women, so that they die in childbirth."[3]

Ergot probably also played an important role in the Greek Mysteries. Albert Hofmann, who discovered LSD, and Richard Schultes wrote: "In an interdisciplinary analysis ... the mysterious rituals of Ancient Greece – an enigma which is four thousand years old, are related to a dazed state which is caused by the parasitic fungus *Claviceps*. Nowadays it is believed that *Claviceps paspali*, and possibly other varieties which take over the plant *Lolium* and other indigenous cereals in Greece, are responsible for the dazed state which form the basis for the ecstasy experienced in the Mysteries."[2]

As the Greeks did not eat rye – because of the ergot, the "black, unpleasant smelling fruit of Thracea and Macedonia"[4] – it disappeared from European history for a long time, and there is no mention of the toxic effect of ergot in Roman pharmaceutical works. It was only with the development of the Christian culture in Europe that rye returned and the first descriptions of the serious consequences of ergot poisoning appeared at the beginning of the Middle Ages.

Widespread epidemics broke out in many parts of Europe; in 1039 there was an epidemic in France in the region of St. Didier-la-Mothe (Dauphiné). A nobleman from this region who was called Gaston, and his son, also succumbed to the dreadful disease. The local church contained the relics of St. Anthony (251–356 AD), a hermit also known as the father of monks, who lived in the Egyptian desert for decades and died at the age of 105. Gaston and his son begged the hermit to save them, and solemnly promised to give him all their worldly wealth if he did so. The miracle happened – they were cured. They built a hospital, and in 1098 a lay order of physicians and knights was founded. In the course of time, this order was to develop to become the new European branch of the militant order of the Brothers of St. Anthony, which had been founded in Egypt and Ethiopia at the end of the fourth century. However, from that time the order's main aim was to help the sick and those who had been made homeless as a result of suffering from the terrible symptoms of the disease caused by ergot poisoning.

How did this disease manifests itself? When the highly toxic grains of ergot were ground into flour with the still unaffected grains of rye and then baked and eaten, this resulted in severe itching and extremely painful burning sensations in the limbs, which eventually turned completely black and cold and then atrophied. (We now known that this gangrenous disease is caused by ergotine, an extremely strong toxin present in ergot. This contracts the smaller peripheral capillaries, and consequently is used in medicine and gynaecology to induce labour and inhibit bleeding.) These terrible sensations of burning and being parched were accompanied by fits, nervous epileptic cramps and delirious states, full of hallucinations. Because of the overwhelming feelings of being on fire, the disease was referred to as "the Holy Fire", "St. Anthony's Fever" or "St. Anthony's Fire".

The descriptions of two chroniclers of that time follow below. The first comes from an official record: "A terrible agony with swollen blisters which devour the body with revolting putrefaction."[4] The monk, Sigbert of Gembloux, wrote: "It was a year of epidemics in which many people who were inwardly consumed by the Holy Fire perished from their rotting limbs, which turned as black as coal. They either died a miserable death, or lived on in even greater misery after their rotten hands and feet had been cut off. However, many people suffered from nervous cramps."[5]

The Brothers of St. Anthony founded their order for these people. On the main roads they built hundreds of hospitals and nursing homes, where people who had been smitten with St. Anthony's Fire – as well as those suffering from other diseases – and people who had been uprooted, could seek refuge.

In those days a cure was seen as a spiritual event. St. Anthony's power manifested itself in the medicinal drinks and remedies which were brought into contact with his relics. The presence of the saint in these relics gave the remedies their power. The sick came to him.

However, he was also present and his powers worked through the overwhelmingly beautiful imagery of the great spiritual works of art which the Brothers of St. Anthony commissioned as therapeutic remedies. Therefore it was traditional for the sick to be brought first to the altar with its paintings and other works of art, in the hope that the powers of St. Anthony, as well as those of Christ, which were in these works, would bring them inner peace and harmony. This also made a physical cure possible – like a miracle – with the supporting medication. However, the cure of the spirit was always the main thing, because disease was viewed as the result of inner weaknesses and faults. Therefore the cure should take place primarily in man's inner self.

One of the altars which was specially made and painted for this purpose is the world famous altar in the Church of the monastic hospital of St. Anthony in Isenheim, situated on the busy pilgrims' way through the Alsace. The Isenheim Altar in Colmar was painted by Matthias Grünewald.

The Isenheim Altar

In this context it is not necessary to describe the whole inner experience of sick people brought before the Isenheim Altar. We are concerned with the effects of ergot, for we are seeking the roots of the LSD experience. Briefly, it was possible for the diseased person to inwardly identify with the realistic and heart-rending image of Christ's crucifixion, so that he was able to experience himself as an eternal spiritual being through other images. He would take in the strength of Christ's resurrection so that he could withstand and conquer his own sickness, and his suffering and the images which tore him apart psychologically. The last painting portrayed the temptation of St. Anthony in the desert; a representation of both the torturing as well as the beneficial forces of the soul of those consumed by St. Anthony's Fire, painted in a realistic as well as artistic way (see the illustration on p. 42).

Photographs overleaf: The Isenheim Altar. 1: The Temptation of St Anthony; 2: St Anthony.

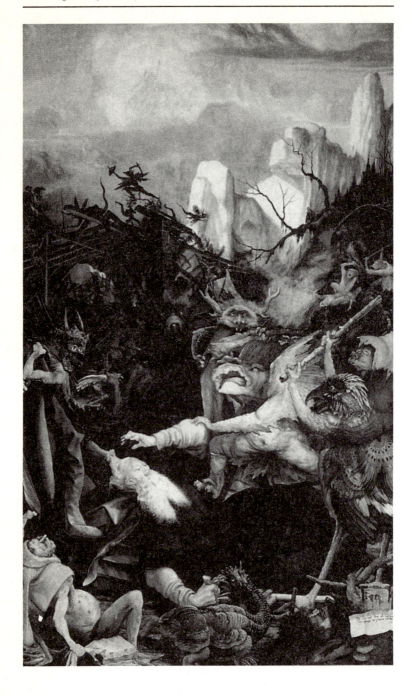

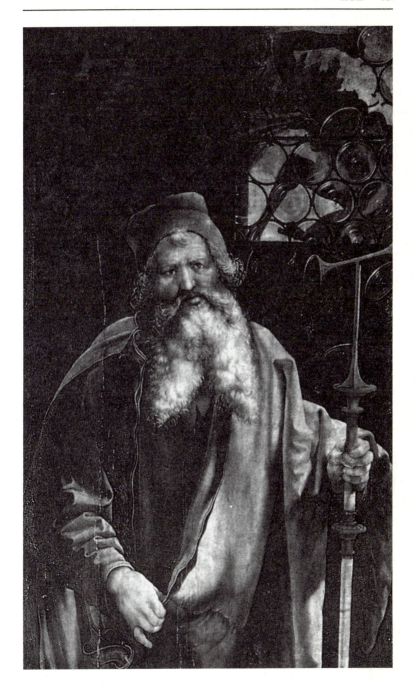

In *Der Isenheimer Altar des Matthias Grünewald,* Gottfried Richter describes this scene as follows: "Directing the gaze to the right-hand panel, this then reveals the completely different terrible scene in which St. Anthony, in his indefatigable battle against the demons, is attacked by them one day, as related by Anastasius. He had challenged them, and they attacked him, destroying his house and setting fire to it, and hitting and kicking down the defenceless. Grünewald painted the impotent man surrendered to his executioners, the house destroyed as a sorry framework, and this nightmare of an orgy of hatred and malicious delight in which the demons are triumphant, with the same cruel realism and the same lack of compassion with which he painted the Crucifixion of the Redeemer.

What courage it took to use this terrible image as the last in the series! How daring! When we imagine someone who had succumbed to this cruel epidemic, and had dragged himself to the altar to seek help so that the power of the painting could have its effect on him, we wonder what he saw. He saw himself. This is how he looked under the mocking grimace of the demon of sickness covered in sores, crouching in the bottom left corner of the painting, surrendered to the oppressive forces of despair and fear, kicked down, broken, shattered. But those who had not been tortured by the disease were also petrified with fear in front of this image. The expression, the gestures, the whole appearance of these terrible figures revealed to them the forces which can be the most dreadful enemies of man: stupidity, insensitivity, brutality, vanity, the dullness of pure physical violence, reptilian lack of soul. Anyone exposed to their raging felt completely abandoned, which also coincided with the experience shown on a note pinned to a tree trunk in the bottom right of the painting: "Ubi eras bone Jhesu? Ubi eras? Quare non affuisti, ut vulnera mea sanares?" (Where were you, good Jesus, where were you? Why were you not here to heal my wounds?)

These words, allegedly spoken by the tortured saint, become the key to the enigma of the whole scene when one realizes that they were not the final words of the story. They were, in those days, responded to with an answer that was certainly known to everyone who came to Isenheim. There was a voice:

"Anthony, I was here, but I waited to watch your struggle. As you stood firm, I will help you in future, and ensure that your name will be honoured everywhere.

When St. Anthony heard this, he stood up to give thanks, and was strengthened so much that he felt how much more strength he had now than he had before ..."

Then the sick person would see that help was on its way. That the heavens had opened, and that the angels were descending to earth, while the demons were cast below. A little longer, and the whole nightmare would be over. Therefore the sick were able to realize that St. Anthony had suffered in the same way.[6]

Because St. Anthony had held out, the sick man – strengthened by the power of the saint through whom the power of Jesus was working – was also able to endure his torments and could hope to be cured without his inner spirit being broken.

In this context we are concerned with the striking correspondence between the "tableau of demons" in the soul of the poisoned victim and the terrifying experience of a bad trip or horror trip which can take place in the soul of someone using LSD. For example: "I can only describe the horror with similar examples. Just imagine being forced to watch helplessly while monsters devour your children. Then increase this emotion a thousand times and it will give you a vague idea of my dreadful experience."[7] In another account someone says: "I hardly recognized the woman next door who brought me milk – in the course of the evening I drank more than two litres. She was no longer Mrs. R., but a malevolent evil witch with an ugly face, distorted with many colours."[8]

In their work, *Handbuch der Rauschdrogen* (Handbook of Hallucinogenic Drugs), Schmidbauer and Vom Scheidt summarized these experiences in the following way: "The most common risk is the bad trip, an acute attack of fear in which the (promised or expected) LSD heaven becomes a hell. The drugged person feels threatened by wild animals or human persecutors, devils and torturers. His sense of reality may collapse, resulting in a short psychotic-like reaction ... If the trip does not wear off, this can be followed by a longer psychotic phase. The victim acts like a madman (usually similar to a case of paranoid hallucinatory schizophrenia) and has to be committed to a psychiatric hospital."[9]

Thus the panel of the Temptation of St. Anthony seems rather like an original version of a bad trip or horror trip.

This brings us to the question posed by Franziska Sarwey in the introduction to her book, *Grünewald-Studien; zur Realsymbolik des Isenheimer Altars* (Grünewald Studies: On the realistic symbolism of the Isenheim Altar):

"Thus the figure of a devil appears above St. Anthony on the right panel of the Isenheim Altar (see top right on illus. 3, opposite p. 00), whose singular horns are actually reminiscent of the ergot fungus on wheat which was responsible for the epidemic of St. Anthony's fire. The devil is breathing out the poisonous fumes."

However, it is now known that the connection between the "holy fire" and contaminated wheat was discovered only at the end of the seventeenth century, while ergot itself was discovered only in the mid-nineteenth century. Thus the question is whether the artistic design was pure coincidence."[10]

Whatever the case, St. Anthony was the salvation of the sick. Prepared and purified by his scores of years as a hermit, he was able to tolerate the venomous stench of the breath of the demonic ergot creature (above his left shoulder) without being affected, with infinite resignation and almost with a smile on his lips, looking into the world and towards the future, unbroken and full of inner strength (see illustration on p.43).

But who is there to help the unprepared person on a bad trip in her terror and panic?

The discovery of LSD

As stated above, the connection between ergot and St. Anthony's Fire was officially discovered only towards the end of the seventeenth century (in 1676) – about five hundred years after the peak of the epidemics. From that time all sorts of hygienic measures were taken to prevent the ergot from being ground into flour together with the grains of rye, with the result that the disease, which had already declined significantly, hardly appeared again. The last big epidemic took place in 1926–1927 in the area between Kasan and the Urals in southern Russia.

The chemical composition of ergot was studied, and it was used as a raw material for the manufacture of many medicines. In 1918, the toxin alkaloid ergotamine was isolated and used as a medicine for migraine. It was also used as a powerful remedy to stop haemorrhaging in childbirth. Other alkaloids from ergot were also used in medicine, geriatric and psychiatric treatment.

In 1938, while he was working on one of the research projects on the medical applications of ergot, Doctor Albert Hofmann, the chief chemist of the large pharmaceutical company Sandoz in Basel, added a diethylamide group to the lysergic acid which had already been isolated from the ergot. Five years later, to be exact, on Friday

16th April 1943, he ingested a small amount of this new substance which he called LSD Lysergic acid diethylamide "by pure chance", probably because some had remained on his fingers. He was suddenly overcome, became very confused and had to go home. When he arrived, the daylight bothered him so much that he closed his eyes and experienced fantastic visions and enormously colourful imagery which lasted for more than two hours. How was this possible? Where did these images come from? Hofmann realized that he had been working all day only with LSD, but that it was impossible for him to have ingested a significant amount. A few days later, on 19 April 1943, he decided to try a real minimum dose, and for this purpose dissolved a quarter of a milligramme of LSD – which subsequently proved to be ten times the effective dose – in some water. He described the results in detail in his diary, and we include this passage in its entirety because we believe that there is a striking correspondence with the inner experiences which are depicted on the Isenheim Altar on the painting of the Temptation of St. Anthony.

"19 April 1943.

"17.00 hours: onset of dizziness, feelings of fear. Visual perception distorted, symptoms of paralysis, attacks of laughter. He continued the diary on 21 April: "Went home on the bike. From 18.00 to approximately 20.00 hours: heaviest crisis (see special report).

"I managed to write down these last words only with the greatest difficulty. It was already clear to me that Lysergic acid diethylamide had been the cause of the strange experience of the previous Friday, because the changes in perception and experience were similar, only much more profound. It was only with the greatest effort that I was able to talk intelligibly, and I asked my laboratory assistant, who was aware of the experiment I was conducting on myself, to accompany me home. On the way home on the bicycle – there was no car available at that time, for during the war cars were reserved for just a few privileged persons – my condition became a cause for some concern. Everything in my field of vision was moving to and fro and was distorted as in a curved mirror. I also had the sense that I was not moving forwards very quickly on my bike, and yet my assistant told me subsequently that we had cycled very fast. When we eventually reached home in one piece, I was just able to ask my assistant to ring the family doctor and to ask the neighbours for milk. Despite my trance-like state of confusion, I was able to think clearly and effectively for short periods – milk as a non-specific, detoxifying remedy. From time to time the dizziness and the feeling of faintness were so strong that I was no longer able to stand up and had to lie down on the sofa. My environment had changed in a terrifying way. Everything in the room turned round, and the familiar objects and furniture assumed grotesque, often threatening forms. They constantly moved about as though they were alive, as though they were filled with inner restlessness. I hardly recognized the woman next door who brought me milk – in the course of the evening I drank more than two litres. It was no longer Mrs. S., but a malevolent, evil witch with a distorted face of many colours. But worse than these grotesque changes in the outside world were the changes which I perceived in myself. All the efforts of my will to prevent the decay of the outside world and to stop myself dissolving seemed to be in vain. A demon had penetrated me and taken possession of my body, my senses and my soul. I jumped up and screamed to be free of him, but fell back onto the sofa, powerless. I had been conquered by the substance with which I had wanted to experiment. This was the demon who triumphed over my will, mocking me. I was overcome by a terrible fear of being mad. I had entered a different world, in another space with another time. My body seemed to have no feeling and no life; it was that of a stranger. Was I dying? Was this the passage to the other side?

"Occasionally I thought that I was outside my body, and then I became fully aware, like an external observer, of the total tragedy of my condition. To die without being able to say goodbye to my family – my wife and our three children had gone to her parents in Lucerne for the day. Would she ever understand that I had not experimented lightly and irresponsibly, but had actually been extremely careful, and that this effect could not have been foreseen in any way? The thought that not only would a young family prematurely lose a father, but also the idea that my work as a scientist doing chemical research which meant so much to me would be broken off, unfinished in the middle of a fruitful and promising project, caused my fear and despair to grow. Meanwhile I was assailed by the bitter irony that it was the Lysergic acid diethylamide which I had introduced to the world that now forced me to leave it. The peak of my despair had already passed when the doctor arrived. My laboratory assistant told him about the experiment on myself because I was not yet able to utter a coherent sentence. After I had tried to draw his attention to my physical condition, which I believed to be fatal, he shook his head, not knowing what to do, because he could not find one abnormal symptom apart from the extremely dilated pupils. My pulse, blood pressure and respiration were all normal. Therefore he did not give me any medicine, but carried me to the bedroom and stayed at my bedside to watch over me. Slowly I returned from the horrible strange world to my familiar everyday reality. The horrors abated and made way for a feeling of joy and gratitude as my normal feelings and thoughts returned, and as the certainly grew that I had definitely escaped the danger of going mad.

"Now I slowly started to enjoy the fabulous play of colours and shapes which continued behind my closed eyelids. Colourful and fantastic patterns changing kaleidoscopically, opening and closing in circles and spirals, showering fountains of colours, reforming and coalescing again, constantly flowing. It was particularly striking how all my acoustic perceptions, such as the sound of a door knocker, or of a car driving past, were trans- lated into visual impressions. Every sound produced a changing image of an appropriate and lively form and colour ..."[11]

The psychedelic revolution

Following the discovery of LSD, the experiments began. Hofmann's colleagues, Stoll and Rothlin, carried out tests on volunteers for four years and then published their results in 1947. As the Sandoz company had started marketing LSD, countless researchers throughout the world were able to do research, and this resulted in more than 600 publications in scientific journals. In the 1950s many experiments were carried out in psychiatry. LSD was used in particular to induce so-called experimental psychoses, and it was hoped that this would give a greater insight into schizophrenic psychosis and its psychotherapeutic treatment.

1961 saw a new approach. In that year a lecturer in psychology at Harvard University (US), who was virtually unknown up to that time, started experimenting with LSD after experiencing the influence of the consciousness changing properties of the psilocybin mushroom and the peyote cactus while on holiday in Mexico the year before. This forty-year-old lecturer, Timothy Leary, regularly took LSD himself, and together with his younger colleague Richard Alpert, started to carry out many experiments with students. Soon an almost religious cult developed around LSD which quickly expanded to become a worldwide youth movement in which the use of consciousness expanding drugs played a central and enormously important role for the first time. The aim was to achieve a higher, ecstatic consciousness, and LSD was the means or sacrament for achieving this.

Leary wrote: "I have repeated this biochemical and (to me) sacramental ritual ... and, almost every time, I have been awed by religious revelations as shattering as the first experience." (In a period of six years he took LSD over 600 times.)"[12] He also wrote: "During a carefully prepared, loving LSD session a woman can have hundreds of orgasms."[13] "The ecstasy was given many names: 'samhadi', 'satori', 'numina', 'nirvana', 'mystical or visionary state', 'transcendentalism' ... For centuries it has been known that the state of ecstasy can be evoked by methods which change the chemical processes within the body – by fasting, contemplative concentration, yoga exercises, and eating foods and drugs. The ecstasy produced by drugs was recently described as 'the psychedelic experience'."[14]

Countless young people went in search of this experience with LSD which he recommended as "the path, the truth and the deity".[14] There was general opposition to this: Sandoz withdrew LSD from the market and ceased production. On 15 July 1965, LSD was prohibited in the United States, and in many countries, including the Netherlands and Germany it was classified under the Opium Act. However, for many young people seeking spiritual enlightenment LSD was like a dream. Preparation and purification were no longer necessary. A "free", ecstatic, spiritual consciousness was up for grabs. This was particularly attractive to a youth which was actually turning away from the one-sided materialism of the consumer society, that was in their eyes in danger of destroying the earth and mankind, and that was seeking another, better world with room for nature and for humankind and its creative imagination.

The establishment and the psychedelic movement (flower power, hippies) were diametrically opposed to each other. The authorities imposed prohibitions and prison sentences. Leary was sentenced in 1966. The youth movement went underground and created a subculture in which LSD and other hallucinogenic drugs (including, to a lesser extent, marijuana/hashish) became the doorway to a world of all-encompassing unity, peace and freedom which later proved illusory.

The possibilities of LSD had been overestimated: too many people succumbed to schizophrenic psychosis after shorter or longer periods, and became paranoid and depressive and alienated from reality. In 1970, Hofmann warned: "The effects of the Mexican hallucinatory mushrooms, which completely change our experience, and in this sense entail unbelievable dangers, explain why these drugs were taboo for so-called primitive people. For them they were sacred drugs, used only by the priest/medicine man in the context of religious ceremonies."[15]

Hofmann continued: "Because there are no longer any taboos in our society, and there is actually a general tendency to remove the remaining inhibitions, all the attempts of officialdom to warn and educate people about the possible dangers of hallucinatory drugs were unfortunately ineffective. Bearing in mind their responsibilities, the manufacturers and the ministry of health could only restrict the use of hallucinatory drugs for scientific research and purely medical applications by imposing strict regulations. Such political measures are not the ideal solution, but in view of the present drug situation in our society, it is the only possible one."[15]

A year later he met Leary, who had just escaped from prison in California and had been granted asylum in Switzerland: "This personal meeting with Leary gave me the impression of an amiable character who was convinced of his mission and who stood up for his views with a sense of humour, but quite uncompromisingly. Convinced as he is of the miraculous effects of psychedelic drugs and the optimism resulting from these, he has his head in the clouds and tends to underestimate or totally ignore the practical difficulties, unpleasant aspects and dangers."[16]

Six months later, in February 1972, they met again. Hofmann wrote: "Leary seemed changed. He made a floating and absent-minded impression."[16] Shortly afterwards, Leary was apprehended at the airport in Kabul in Afghanistan, taken back to America and returned to prison in California. Following a much publicized trial he was sentenced to fifteen years imprisonment for setting up a gigantic trade in all sorts of drugs. For example, the equipment for producing fourteen million LSD trips was discovered. Leary, who had started to call himself the High Priest and Reincarnation of Jesus Christ[17] promised to reform, and was released fairly quickly in the spring of 1976. Three years later, Hofmann wrote about him: "From his friends I heard that he is now concerned with the psychological problems of space travel and is doing research into cosmic patterns in the stars which correspond to the human nervous system. In other words, he is studying problems with which the government probably will not interfere."[18]

As for Hofmann himself, he gave an interview in 1979 on his "child",

LSD. "Because LSD has been used lightly, which does not suit the nature of its effects, because it has been used on the drug scene to replace stimulants, there have been many accidents and catastrophes which have given LSD a general reputation of being a satanic drug ... Special inner and external preparations are necessary for an LSD experiment to be a meaningful experience. Its wrongful and illegal use has made LSD a heavy burden of responsibility to me."[19] In the same year he summarized his work in his book *LSD: My Problem Child* at the age of seventy-three, i.e. almost forty-two years after producing LSD in 1938: "Meditation is a preparation for the same goal as that aimed for and achieved in the Mysteries of Eleusis. It is conceivable that in the future LSD could be used to a greater extent to achieve the Enlightenment which crowns meditation. For me, the real significance of LSD is the possibility of supporting meditation aimed at the mystical experience of a higher and, at the same time, deeper reality of the material aspect of life ... This use is entirely in accordance with the essence and nature of the effect of LSD as a sacred drug."[20]

The effects of LSD

We should start by introducing several concepts which we consider essential for understanding the effect of LSD (as well as other drugs). These concepts belong to the spiritual science of anthroposophy. They are related to the human organism.

In spiritual terms, human beings are composed of a visible part (more accurately, the part that can be perceived with the senses), and an invisible part (which cannot be perceived with the senses).

The following elements can be distinguished:
- The physical body, i.e. the externally visible principle which can be weighed, and which human beings have in common with minerals.
- The ethereal body (also known as the living body), i.e. the whole of the living processes as expressed, for example, in growth and reproduction, which ensures that the physical body does not fall apart until the moment of death. Human beings have this in common with plants.
- The astral body, which is the carrier of consciousness, such as perceptions, passions, instincts, drives, feelings, impulses of the will (but also of all the thoughts which pass through our soul every day). Human beings have an astral body in common with animals;
- The Self, which means that human beings are the crown of

creation and that we are conscious of ourselves (self-awareness).

In the waking state these four parts of each person are constantly relating to each other and interreacting. A more detailed description of this concept of human beings is given below.

We have seen that LSD, which is prepared from ergot – which is toxic – is itself a toxic substance, and causes extremely far-reaching changes in consciousness when a tiny amount is taken. What is the explanation for this? To find an answer to this question we should first concern ourselves in a more general sense with the effect of toxins on the human organism.

What happens when we ingest a fatal amount of poison? Obviously we die. In terms of the division of man's body into its different parts, death means that the ethereal body leaves the physical body, and that only this physical body remains on earth as a corpse. Life withdraws from it and the ethereal body is separated from the physical body. The connection between these two parts of the body is broken. People who have almost died or who appear to have died are familiar with this process from their own experience, and are often able to describe it subsequently, as in this example: "However, suddenly Mrs. Schwarz saw herself sliding slowly and calmly out of her body, and soon she was floating a little way above her bed. With a great sense of humour she told us how she could look down at the bodies stretched out below her, looking pale and disgusting. She felt a great sense of astonishment and surprise, but was not frightened or anxious."[21] This is taken from Elisabeth Kübler-Ross's book, *On Death and Life Afterwards*, in which she collected many experiences of people who had consciously experienced the process in which the ethereal body leaves the physical body. She concluded: "After collecting countless cases over so many years, we can come to the conclusion that in all the experiences in a life-threatening situation, when one is floating on the edge of death, the following facts can be considered to be the common denominator. At the moment of death we will all experience the separation of our essential immortal self from its temporary home, i.e. the physical body. This immortal self is also known as the soul. In symbolic terms, this Self which liberates itself from the earthly body, can be compared to a butterfly crawling out of its cocoon – an image which appeals to children. As soon as we have left our physical body, we realize that we are not affected by any trace of panic, fear or anxiety. We always feel that we are "whole" and unviolated. We are completely conscious of the spot where the accident or the death took place, whether it was in a hospital or our own bedroom that we had a heart attack, or it may also be the spot where a car accident happened, or an airplane crash. For example, we can clearly see which people belong to the resuscitation team, or see all the people who came running up to free a wounded or injured body from the wreck of a car. We can observe all this from a few yards away without being really involved mentally. I deliberately use the term "mentally", because in most cases we are no longer able to use our physical mental faculties or brain at those moments. Usually these experiences take place when the encephalogram no longer gives any reading, or when the doctors cannot find any signs of life. At the moment when we experience the scene of our own death, we can hear the conversations of the bystanders observing all the details. We can see how they are dressed, and know what they are thinking, though without this experience having any negative quality. The second body in which we are temporarily accommodated, and which we experience as such, is not a physical but an ethereal body."[22]

What is the connection with the effect of LSD? People who use LSD are also able to have this experience of near death, of the ethereal body moving out of the physical body for a while. The first person to take LSD, Albert Hofmann, described this as follows: "Sometimes I had the feeling that I was standing outside my own body. I thought I had died. My 'ego' was floating somewhere in space, and I saw my body lying dead on the sofa."[23]

Timothy Leary wrote: "I understood that I had died, that I – Timothy Leary – the naive, carefree Timothy Leary was dead. I turned around and saw my body lying on the bed."[24]

Fortunately these two users were not really dead, but they had left their physical body. Their ethereal body had separated itself from the physical body, but not for good. In other words, they had died temporarily. Because experiences of a physical body are possible while the LSD is still working, which shows that the ethereal body is still partly connected to the physical body, this can be described even more precisely: the use of LSD results in a *partial* death.[25] The ethereal body partly separates from the physical body; the toxin partly tears us away from our physical body – even if only a minute quantity is taken (even 0.00003 grammes is sufficient for a powerful reaction) – and we enter the realms of the dead.

This phenomenon is of the greatest importance for understanding the effect of LSD and the other mind-expanding drugs, viz., that as a result of using these toxins we die a little bit, making a start on the process of leaving the body or dying. In this process of dying, which is on the way to death, other experiences await us which people who have almost died, or who were apparently dead, also experienced and which they have reported. Timothy Leary went on to write: "My life ended for me. Once again I experienced the many events which I had long forgotten."[24]

We certainly often hear about this cinematic end to the panorama of life in the descriptions of people who have used LSD. Life is experienced as a panorama or in flashes or isolated moments, for example, the earliest years of childhood or even birth, sometimes in a way that is easy to comprehend, or sometimes chaotically, but always in a very lively way. Comparing this with the experience of people who have almost died or who appear to have died, a striking correspondence appears. Here is one account which illustrates this: "In Vietnam I was wounded and "died", although I constantly remained completely conscious of what was happening to me. I was hit by six rounds of machine-gun fire ... At the moment that I was hit, my life started to pass before me like a film; it was as though my whole life, from the time that I was a baby, passed in front of me in images. I could remember everything. The images were extremely vivid and clear. My life flashed past, from my earliest memories to my most recent ones, and all this happened very quickly."[26] In his book, *Life after this life: experiences of people during their clinical death*, Raymond Moody summarizes these experiences of looking back over the life that is past, as follows: "This look back is a succession of memories, though of a very special sort. In the first place, it takes place extremely quickly. When the memories are described in terms of time, they are described as succeeding each other very rapidly in chronological order. Other people do not remember this sort of chronological order at all. For them the memories are like a single take in which they saw everything at once, observing everything at a glance. Either way, everyone seems to agree that in terms of real time the experience lasts only a minute."[27]

Elisabeth Kübler-Ross confirmed these experiences with the help of Victor Fränkl's research: "A few decades ago, when there was still hardly any interest in these subjects, he was collecting information in Europe on mountaineers who had fallen, and who, in the face of death, had seen their whole lives passing before them like a film. He checked to find out how much of their lives they had seen passing in their mind's eye in the few seconds of their fall. Then he came to the conclusion that during this sort of out-of-the-body experience, time as such cannot exist. Many people have had exactly the same experience just before drowning or in other life-threatening situations."[28]

How is this possible and how can it be explained? In his book, *The Science of the Secrets of the Soul*, Rudolf Steiner also described these phenomena in detail, and explained that the ethereal body could be largely separated from the physical body momentarily, for example, after a great shock, with the result that the ethereal forces which are liberated enter consciousness (the astral body), so that the content of the memory which is in the ethereal body is transformed into *images*. According to Rudolf Steiner, it is the ethereal body which carries our memories and stores all the impressions we have gathered during our lives. Everything which is apparently forgotten is stored – unforgotten – in the ethereal body. When we die, the ethereal body completely separates from the physical body, with the result that the entire content of the memory can suddenly blossom in the astral body, so that we can survey our past life in a large inner panorama. The ethereal body no longer has to give form to the physical body, and can therefore place all its forces at the disposal of the astral body, where they can be turned into images, i.e. the image of a past life.

This also happens to a greater or lesser extent to someone who uses LSD. As a result of the partial death experienced by the user, all sorts of contents from the memory which had already been long forgotten can be turned into inner images. This consciousness of impressions from the ethereal body can go back a long way; it can contain impressions from a long time ago, such as those going back before birth, and even before conception. In this last case, the impressions are those which were made on that part of the ethereal body which is inherited from parents.[29] In their turn, they were in the ethereal flow of inherited memories from their parents, great-grandparents, and so on, which enables us to look at the increasingly general memory of mankind, i.e. the history of the creation of the human organism.

With regard to foetal memories, Timothy Leary wrote: "I also experienced my past as a history of development; I experienced my evolution until I recognized myself as a single cell organism. All this transcended the bounds of my reason."[14] These, and similar experiences of Timothy Leary, were confirmed by the large-scale research of Stanislav Grof, who analyzed more than 3,800 LSD sessions, and came to the conclusion that foetal, embryonic, ancestral, racial, collective and evolutionary experiences played an important role in the inconceivably large range of different LSD experiences.[30]

The area of the collective unconscious and its archetypes (Jung) is thus made accessible by the effects of LSD; in fact, Jung had always warned against this – quite independently from the use of drugs – when he referred to "psychic inflation", a phenomenon in which the unconscious reigns supreme and the individual and what she comprises is overwhelmed until, in an extreme case, the individual becomes psychotic or ultimately destroys herself.

In addition, he warned that "approaching the unconscious led to an increasing degree of social isolation. Gradually the autonomy of unconscious figures increases to such an extent that it results in aggression and real fear." (1944)[31] We will return to these and other dangers of the use of LSD later on.

If we restrict ourselves to life between birth and death, it is striking that it is not only images, but also feelings and aspects of a strong emotional nature that can be brought into consciousness by LSD. This also applies to repressed and forgotten events with a strong content of fear or emotion, i.e. to traumas which can result in lengthy depressions, neuroses and other forms of disturbed behaviour. This also explains why LSD is sometimes used in psychotherapy, although there is a danger that the sudden strong consciousness of this sort of unprocessed content can lead to severe feelings of fear and panic attacks in the patient. In the Netherlands, the work of Professor Bastiaans is well known in this respect. He gave LSD to people suffering from a so-called "concentration camp syndrome". The experiences of the concentration camp which had been repressed were brought back to consciousness with the use of LSD. It was then possible to treat them with psychotherapy. (We do not give any opinion about this form of psychotherapy here – we are merely concerned with the effects of LSD.) This example also shows that LSD is able to separate the ethereal body partly from the physical body, independently of the will, with the result that this ethereal body and the images and emotions contained in it become perceptible to us. We will now examine this in more detail.

In Rudolf Steiner's descriptions, this ethereal body is not described as a regular ethereal organism, but as a very complicated tissue comprised of four different sorts of ethereal principles which permeate each other and work together to maintain and give form to the physical body. The question arises whether these four different sorts of ethereal principles can also be recognized in the descriptions of the experiences of people who use LSD.

To find the answer to this question, we will describe each of these four ethereal principles in the words of Bernard Lievegoed in his book, *Mens op de drempel* (*Man on the Threshold*). Then we will compare this with accounts of LSD users, or with the specialist literature, for each ethereal quality.

1.   Ethereal form

Bernard Lievegoed: "(The ethereal form) is also known as ethereal crystallization or ethereal life. The rhythms of this ethereal quality create the geometric order of matter in crystal formations. Ethereal form has a rigidifying effect. The Snow Queen in Anderson's fairytale is an appropriate symbol of this force, because everything which touches her becomes motionless.[32]

LSD experience: "I saw some splendid multicolored geometric patterns ..."[33]

The specialist literature also contains many visual descriptions of luminescent formations, networks, cobwebs, snowflakes or benzol-like ring structures (a particular chemical compound).[34]

2.   Chemical ether

Bernard Lievegoed: "Chemical ether or sound ether creates order in matter in the liquid element. The combination and disintegration of endless series of chemical compounds and conversions characterize this ethereal effect in the metabolism ... in the liquid organism."[35]

The specialist literature often refers to the flow and coalescence of colours and sparks, to fountains of colours, sparkling bubbles of liquid and raging whirlpools."[36] However, chemical ether is not usually seen in its pure form, but permeated with experiences of light and colour (forces of ethereal light) see 3 below.

These experiences – particularly visual experiences – of the endlessly changing luminescent and colourful eddies in the element of water, the combination and dissolution of liquid flows, including the air bubbles contained in them, were the basis of the light shows which were popular at the start of the psychedelic era. In these shows, the flow of liquid was projected on a large screen during pop concerts to support and reinforce the musical experience. It would be difficult to conceive of a more striking externalized image of sound ether than this combination of externally projected flows of liquid and externally audible sounds.

3. Ethereal light

Bernard Lievegoed: "Ethereal light, which could also be called ethereal consciousness. Consciousness takes place in the rhythms of ethereal light, and as such, these rhythms form the link with the next organizational principle, the astral level. In this context the central area of operation is the nervous/sensory system."[35]

LSD experience: "When a friend put on a record by Telemann, the whole world of my perceptions changed as though a magic wand had been waved. The whole of space was filled with a blinding white light, like that of burning magnesium. This phenomenon seemed to extend into infinity."[37]

The perception of this quality of ethereal light is so general, permeating everything when LSD is taken, that it is virtually always referred to with great emphasis in the specialist literature. The *Handbuch der Rauschdrogen* (The Handbook of Hallucinatory Drugs) states: "Almost everyone will describe the increased brightness of colours as the first sign of the psychological change. All perceptions are more intense, with more light, and the colours are more saturated."[38]

Van Ree wrote: "The changes in perception are particularly strong in the visual field. The greater intensity of the experience of colour is particularly striking."[39] Van Epen wrote: "The beginning of the trip is usually characterized by changes in perception. Grass is greener than usual, the sky is bluer. All the colours and forms are charged with a high degree of intensity; it is as though everything assails the tripper more intensely, and he feels and experiences them more deeply... Sometimes all sorts of things radiate light."[40]

How can this be explained? As described above, the ethereal forces are partly separated from the physical body as a result of the effect of LSD. When this concerns forces of ethereal light which become separated from particular organs of the physical body (as described in greater detail below), and when these forces of ethereal light then connect with the quality of ethereal light already present in our senses, we become conscious of this intensified activity of light in our astral body, and this results in a more intense experience of light and colour.

This can be illustrated with the following example: if you look at a red dot on a piece of white paper without interruption for one minute, and then turn away to focus the gaze on the white paper next to it, a luminous spot of green will appear on the white paper.

Why is this? By looking at the red dot for one minute a significant process of disintegration takes place in the retina. This is restored by the ethereal body, and the forces of ethereal light which restore it are perceived as a red after-image, i.e. as the shining green spot (the complementary colour of red). We are actually perceiving the forces of ethereal light; the green dot does not physically exist on the white paper.

Just as this after-image is produced by the impression of the restorative forces of ethereal light, in our visual/sensory conscious-ness (astral body), the vibrant perceptions of light and colour are caused by the impression of the ethereal forces of light released by LSD in the same consciousness, where they may or may not be combined with ordinary sensory impressions. This can be explained as follows. When the eyes are closed, the astral body is able to perceive the "extra" ethereal light in a pure form; when the eyes are open, the astral body combines this ethereal light with ordinary visual/perceptual impressions resulting in the above-mentioned in-tensified experiences of light and colour, or otherwise it projects the ethereal light on the surrounding world of perception in the form of hallucinations in a way that is characteristic of the astral body.

Van Ree described one of his own experiences by way of example: "A few months later I took another LSD trip somewhere else. Once again everywhere was filled with colourful visions, this time without any accompanying music. Then my wife came into the room. At the moment she came in, the same bright white light started to shine from her hair, which shone like gold. It was as though it was full of lace work sewn with gold and silver thread. I never saw my wife looking as beautiful as she did then."[37]

These hallucinations of light (and colour) are very common with the use of LSD. We will return to this later.

Finally, it should be mentioned in this context that LSD users can have severe problems with this excessive stimulation of ethereal light. For example, Hofmann was hardly able to bear ordinary daylight during his first trip, and this is why wearing sunglasses (tripping glasses) was all the rage when LSD first became popular.

4.   Ethereal heat

Bernard Lievegoed: "The effect of ethereal heat permeates the whole organism. The central organ is present in the circulation of the blood, and ethereal heat is the medium through which man's spiritual self can come into contact with the living physical body."[35]

There is very little mention of the release of the forces of spiritual heat in the specialist literature on LSD; this is the domain of opium, morphine and heroin, particularly when they are injected into the bloodstream.

Nevertheless, there are some exceptions. One of the people living at Arta wrote about his LSD experiences: "I took LSD for the first time when I was about eighteen. I felt good, and my whole body glowed, but nothing else happened. As I was looking for more, I continued to take it. Often I took twice or three times the dose taken by my friends, but the feeling remained the same, a sense of well-being and a glowing body."

A summary of the points described above and an examination of the extent to which each of the four ethereal principles are released from the physical body by the effect of LSD clearly shows that it is above all ethereal light, and to a lesser extent chemical ether (sound ether), and to an even lesser extent ethereal life, that is separated from the physical body by the effect of this drug. With regard to ethereal heat, this only happens in exceptional cases.

With regard to the question of where this happens in the physical body, the following fact is of great importance: tests with radioactive LSD show that after being taken orally in the usual way, LSD is deposited particularly in the liver and kidneys (and to a very limited extent, in the brain).[41] It is then excreted within a period of eight to twelve hours.[42] According to the anthroposophical study of man, the liver is the centre of ethereal sound, while the kidneys are the centre of ethereal light. Therefore it should not come as any surprise that it is these two ethereal qualities which are perceived, as they are separated from their main physical base, i.e. their physical organic centre, as a result of the effect of the toxic LSD. Therefore the liver and the kidneys die off to a significant extent when LSD is used; these organs are poisoned so that they break down, releasing ethereal forces, resulting in the experiences which are caused in particular by the extra ethereal light, and to a lesser extent, the extra ethereal sound.

In addition, recent scientific research shows that LSD also affects the *metabolic* processes in certain parts of the nervous system. LSD affects the transfer of stimuli from one nerve cell (neuron) to another – which takes place by means of certain substances (so-called neuro-transmitters) – by affecting the neuro-transmitter serotonin. This is because LSD stimulates the serotonin receptors in the receptor nerve cells.[43] The cells of these serotonin neurons are in the brain*stem*, and send their nerve ends to many parts of the brain, such as the cortex, the limbic system (related to emotional life) and to other brain centres which regulate, amongst other areas, the sensory area.

Thus LSD brings about changes in the serotonin-secreting nervous system with the result that forces of ethereal light are also released here. This can result in hallucinations. Rudolf Steiner discussed this in a lecture on 21 March 1918: "Imagine that one of man's cognitive organs is affected by abnormal conditions ... In that case, he could not surrender to the perceptions received from the outside world independently of the forces of growth, digestion and metabolism (i.e. the ethereal forces), and he would have hallucinations and visions ... Things which should serve completely different processes enter consciousness and the field of visual perception. That is why hallucinations and visions are always an expression of the fact that there is something in the person concerned that is not right."[44] Thus the release of the forces of ethereal light also takes place in the brain-stem, i.e. in that part of the nervous system regarding which, Olaf Koob, a follower of Rudolf Steiner, wrote: "It is responsible for all the dreamlike instinctive faculties which create images, and it is reminiscent of a period of development when man still possessed an instinctive, hazy clairvoyance."[45] (Also see *Return to the Gods*, pp. 17–20.)

With regard to the strong effect which LSD has on the liver and the kidneys, it is easy to understand that the experiences brought about in the soul by the effect of the drug have a strong emotional character and influence the feelings. This is because, according to the anthroposophical science of man, the liver is the foundation and ethereal memory of our feelings, while the kidneys fulfil this function for the emotions. Therefore when these organs are poisoned, the ethereal forces released in this way evoke more feelings and emotions than we normally have. On the one hand these feelings and emotions can go back to the past, such as cherished childhood memories, as well as oppressed traumas, but, on the other hand, the direct perceptions are also coloured by this component of feelings and emotions during the LSD experience. All thoughts and perceptions are permeated with feelings and emotions.

There is more to it than this. It is precisely because the liver and kidneys are poisoned that a situation develops which is described in anthroposophical psychiatry as being characteristic of psychosis. In other words, ethereal forces which normally permeate the organs of the human body are separated from these organs and are forced into consciousness (astral body). The use of LSD artificially produces a condition of temporary liver and kidney psychosis. Hopefully, as soon as the drug has finished working, the ethereal forces which were released can find their way back to the organs damaged by the poison. If this is not the case, and the delicate structure of the organs has been damaged too specifically, it can result in a long-term psychotic condition.

What is a liver psychosis? Lievegoed describes this, inter alia, in the following terms: "... Strange visions and hallucinations occur in relation to reality. Crossing the boundaries in this way can lead to violent reactions, and absurd hallucinations can result. Voices which give orders, or the influence of electric shock waves, are experienced at the same time as being real and not real. This is because the voices and so on are actually heard and experienced, while at the same time the intellect knows that they are not real. When this last support also collapses, the user is generally considered to have gone mad. (An hallucination is the reflection of an organ of the ethereal body in the astral body. As a result of the reflection, there is a consciousness of the organ's function. This reflection disturbs the normal pattern of sickness.) The nature of the hallucinations ... is always in some way related to the user's own biography... Someone with an anxious, obsessive character will have different hallucinations and delusions from someone who naturally enjoys life."[46]

Lievegoed's observation will certainly be recognized by the LSD user. This is clear from Hofmann's description of his hallucinations during his first deliberate trip: "Then I gradually started to enjoy the fabulous play of colours and shapes which took place behind my closed eyelids. Colourful and fantastic patterns changing kaleidoscopically, opening and closing in circles and spirals, showering fountains of colours, reforming and coalescing again, constantly flowing."[47]

In this quotation, Hofmann gives a particularly good description of the visual experience of a liver psychosis. In other words, of the experience which the chemical ethereal forces released from the liver, permeated with the forces of ethereal light from the kidneys, produce in the astral body.

How can we describe a kidney psychosis? In his book, *Die Entwicklung der Seele im Lebenslauf* (The development of the soul through life), the psychiatrist, Rudolf Treichler, describes kidney psychosis as an essentially schizophrenic psychosis which he characterizes as follows: "Three main forms of schizophrenic psychosis can be distinguished. If changes in perception and thinking are in the foreground, this can be described as a paranoid, hallucinatory form of schizophrenia (accompanied by delusions and hallucinations). If the changes are more closely related to the emotions, so that the feelings become stuck, with stupid or childlike behaviour, the condition is diagnosed as 'hebephrenia', with an extremely clear increase in adolescent symptoms. When the symptoms reveal themselves particularly in the will and the patient's motor behaviour, the disease is diagnosed as 'catatonia'. This results in conditions of tension and relaxation, and in rages and paralysis (stupor)."[48]

In his book, *De drugs van de wereld, de wereld van de drugs* (Drugs of the world, the world of drugs), the psychiatrist J.H. van Epen reveals a very clear connection between schizophrenic psychosis and LSD psychosis: "As we have seen, it is possible to become psychotic after the use of LSD, with a state of confusion, anxiety and hallucinations. In most victims this psychosis disappears after a few days or weeks, with or without treatment, but some remain confused for months or years, even without taking LSD again ..."

"The long-term psychoses which can occur after using LSD are usually remarkably similar to schizophrenia. The patients are confused, which becomes immediately obvious when you try to talk to them. Their stories contain strange and illogical elements. They often jump from one subject to another and are unable to focus their attention on a single subject. There are usually hallucinations: they hear 'voices' which say all sorts of things, give orders and respond to their thoughts. Sometimes there are also hallucinations of feelings: vibrations, peculiar sensations and feelings in the stomach and sexual organs, or in the brain. In an LSD psychosis there may be delusions, usually delusions of persecution. The patients feel they are being followed, threatened. The police are observing them; their lives are in danger. This can result in a high level of fear, and sometimes the patients can be extraordinarily aggressive to their imagined attackers. In addition, many of the symptoms of the acute LSD state survive permanently. The patient sees bright colours and dark, sombre outlines around objects which make undulating or rhythmic movements. Sometimes patients are aware of the unhealthy nature of their condition and explain that they have 'become stuck in a trip'.

"It is understandable that most people suffering from chronic LSD psychosis end up in psychiatric institutions where they can hardly be distinguished from other schizophrenic patients. In schizophrenia, confusion, delusions and hallucinations are also common. It is difficult to find reliable criteria which can be used to distinguish the two conditions."[49]

A summary of the above-mentioned points and a comparison of kidney psychosis, schizophrenic psychosis and LSD psychosis, as described by Treichler and Van Epen, leads to the conclusion that the use of LSD results in a temporary kidney psychosis. Because of the hallucinations, confusion and possible delusions accompanying this, this condition is very similar to the paranoid hallucinatory form of schizophrenia. Furthermore, there is a danger that this schizophrenic, psychotic condition can become long-term, so that the ex-LSD user ends up by becoming a psychiatric patient.

Reviewing the above suggests that the use of LSD separates the ethereal forces – in particular ethereal light, to a lesser extent (chemical) sound ether, to an even lesser extent ethereal life, and, very rarely, ethereal heat – from the physical body. This has many far-reaching consequences, of which the following have been mentioned:

a. The experience of a partial death, as expressed in the experience of the departure of the physical body and the reviewing of life up to that moment (or episodes in that life).

b. The experience of foetal, embryonic, ancestral, racial, collective and evolutionary experiences, as the memory content of the ethereal body is released and blossoms in the astral body.

c. The release of strong feelings and emotions due to the separation of the ethereal body, particularly in the liver and kidneys. These colour not only the images in the memory, but also present perceptions and observations.

d. Perceptions and observations are overwhelmed by the qualities of ethereal light which separate from their centre in the kidneys, and then connect with the whole of the sensory and nervous system, particularly the sense of sight.

e. The hallucinations and visions caused by the release of the forces of ethereal light in the serotonin part of the nervous system, in particular in the brain stem. These are a memory of man's former consciousness.

f. A temporary psychotic condition which may be accompanied by hallucinations, confusion and delusions, which, if the condition persists, has all the characteristics of a schizophrenic (paranoid hallucinatory) psychosis.

Before continuing with a more detailed exploration of the question as to what happens to the released ethereal forces, we will first discuss two consequences of the partial separation of the ethereal body which could shed some light on some of the LSD user's important experiences.

a. When the ethereal forces are released and combine, inter alia, with the senses, virtually every LSD user finds that her sensory perceptions become more intense. Sensory impressions are increasingly brought into the astral body – i.e. into consciousness – so that sensory stimuli which had been imperceptible before, now result in perceptions.

    This accounts for the unbelievable experiences which can occur, such as the following: "My senses had become so acute that I could hear someone breathing in the neighbours' house, and I could smell someone making a pudding miles away."[50] George Harrison, guitarist with the Beatles, who started taking LSD in 1967, said: "It was as though I had never before really tasted, spoken, seen, thought or listened."[51]

b. Another experience which is familiar to virtually everyone who has taken LSD is the way in which sensory impressions flow together, the so-called synaesthesia. This was mentioned in the description of Albert Hofmann's first deliberate LSD experience: "It was particularly striking how all my acoustic perceptions, such as the sound of a door knocker, or of a car driving past, were translated into visual impressions. Every sound produced a changing image of a suitable and lively form and colour ..."[52]

Van Epen summarized this phenomenon as follows: "It is worth mentioning the occurrence of so-called 'synaesthetic' perceptions; the intermingling of sensory qualities. For example, music is 'seen', a photograph or landscape can be 'heard', and so on. The tripper may attempt to explain to the outsider that the normal distinction between the senses of sight, hearing, feeling, smell, taste and so on is actually senseless and that, in reality, there is a total experience of visual, acoustic and other perceptions."[53]

Van Ree himself had the following experiences when he used LSD: "Sitting at a table with my chin resting in the palms of my hands, I gazed attentively at the colourful 'Northern lights', hallucinations which played in space in front of me. Gradually I became aware that every sound in the room affected the image. When anyone talked to me, the rhythm of his words became visible in the movements of the veils of colour before me, and sometimes the images of his words actually formed in space in light pastel blues. Feeling the hard, smooth tabletop made the colours appear brighter and more metallic, while stroking the soft fabric of the cloth on the middle of the table transformed the veils into woolly, coloured clouds all around me. So it was as though I could see other people's words, as well as my own sense of touch in space. It was as though the senses of touch, hearing and sight made contact and flowed together."[54]

How can this be explained? We mentioned above that the ethereal body is not a regular ethereal organism, but a very complicated tissue consisting of four different sorts of ethereal principles which are interwoven and interact to maintain and give form to the physical body. In his work, *Science of the Secrets of the Soul*, Rudolf Steiner described it in the first instance as follows: "For the time being, it is sufficient to say that the ethereal body penetrates the physical body everywhere and can be viewed as a sort of architect of the physical body. The form and shape of organs are maintained by the movement and flow of the ethereal body. There is an 'ethereal heart' which serves as the basis for the physical heart, 'an ethereal brain' for the physical brain, and so on. The ethereal body is actually organized like the physical body, but in a more complicated way, and all the living elements intermingle, while the physical body contains separate parts."[55]

The last sentence is particularly important for our study because it reveals that the limits between the functions of the four different sorts of ethereal principle cannot be sharply defined. Because of this, the ethereal forces released by the effect of LSD connect with the senses in several places so that a stimulus in one sensory area also evokes responses, and therefore perceptions, in the other senses. "I tried to tell the others how beautiful it was, but the words came out of my mouth dripping with moisture, or they tasted of colours ... I felt terrible, and in the end I was no longer able to talk, but dropped to the floor, shut my eyes, and the music physically assimilated me. I could smell and touch and feel the music just as much as I could hear it."[56]

Several senses are stimulated by the extra forces of ethereal light (consciousness) which are released; the stimulation of one sense immediately evokes "responses" or sensations in other senses, because the ethereal body works in several places and is potentially present everywhere. Even slight stimulation of just one of the senses immediately evokes reactions in the ethereal bodies of the other senses because of the presence of extra ethereal forces. The astral body connected to these senses then translates the stimulation into sensory perceptions.

Losing the boundaries

Thus the effect of the toxic LSD is to punch a "hole" between the physical body and the ethereal body. The drug pulls these two parts of the person apart, and part of the ethereal body leaves the physical body. As the astral body and the Self are still connected with the entire ethereal body – i.e. also with the part which has become separated – the user is able to experience the impressions of the ethereal body in the outside world and in herself in a conscious way. However, these impressions are usually distorted, as explained in more detail below.

Someone who takes LSD breaks through the boundary to the ethereal world, and does so with violence. She is forcing the door, flying across the threshold, and arrives completely unprepared in an area which is normally entered only by those who have prepared for this for many years. Rudolf Steiner describes that to enter this ethereal world without any danger and be able to make distinctions, years of training are necessary to develop, for example, a clear judgment, patience, the ability to concentrate, a sober and realistic approach, and other spiritual powers. Insofar as one can express this in ordinary language, he describes how it is possible to experience crossing the boundary from the physical world to the ethereal world: "You feel surrounded by thunderstorms on virtually every side. You hear peals of thunder and see flashes of lightning. You know that you are in the room of a house. You feel permeated with a strength hitherto unknown. Then you think you see cracks in the walls around you. You feel obliged to tell yourself or the person you believe to be next to you, that something very serious is happening, that lightning is flashing through the house, that it is shooting down at you and that you are being hit by lightning. It dissolves you."[57]

This could be compared to the following LSD experience described by John Cashman: "The dimensions of the room were changing, now sliding into a fluttering diamond shape, then straining into an oval shape ... Then in a flash of insight I realized to my horror that the black thing (which I saw) was actually devouring me. I was the flower and this foreign, creeping thing was eating me! ... I felt myself dissolving into the terrible apparition, my body melting in waves into the core of blackness, my mind stripped of ego and life and, yes, even death. In one great crystal instant I realized that I was immortal."[58]

There is a striking similarity between these two descriptions. Elsewhere, John Cashman described the following experience: "I saw the most horrible, slimy snake I have ever seen. It was large and ugly and it curled around me ... I knew the snake was swallowing me, bit by bit ... I was becoming a part of it."[59] He also wrote: "I looked up at a seagull, and suddenly it devoured me, as though my existence was sucked up by its eyes."[60]

There are many more examples; these are all experiences in which the consciousness of the LSD user "expands", dissolves, becomes one with part of the world around her. (This is why the term "consciousness-expanding" drugs is used.) It is obvious that for an unprepared and unsuspecting LSD user this can result in terrible fears and panic (known as a "bad trip" or horror trip).

However, it should be remembered that Rudolf Steiner always stressed that, because of the necessity of using terms relating to the physical/sensory world, his description could be no more than an approach or an image for the events which take place in the ethereal world, while the experiences of LSD users often take the form of dream images which arise because the partly separated ethereal body, the astral body and the self are still connected to the senses of the physical body. Because of this connection to the physical senses, all the impressions entering the astral body – in this case, from the ethereal world – which become conscious there, will take the form of images and perceptions from the physical/sensory world, just as they do in dreams (colours, shapes, distances, movements, sounds etc.).

However, in this context, the essential thing is that the ethereal body partly dissolves into (part of) the surrounding world because of the effect of LSD. This results in the experience that the boundaries between the inner world and the outer world disappear. The user is devoured, digested, dissolved, i.e. the ethereal body becomes one with (part of) the surrounding world, and the astral body translates this, in a way that is characteristic for every individual, into waking dream images which represent this process of the separation, evaporation and dissolving of the ethereal body.

The following quotations from various LSD users show that this process of being united with the environment can also be a much more pleasant experience, with an enjoyment of the blurring of the boundaries, the intermingling of the world around, and becoming one with nature: "I was delighted to see that my skin was dissolving in tiny particles and floating away. I felt as though my outer shell was disintegrating and the 'essence' of me was being liberated to join the 'essence' of everything else about me."[61]

"I no longer knew what was real and what was unreal. Was I the table, the book or the music, or was I part of all of it? But it didn't matter much, because whatever I was, I was fantastic."[50]

"I could feel the room in me and I became part of the room. I even 'knew' that everything outside the room, the flowers in the garden, pulsated along with me just as I pulsated along with everything. I felt that I was one with all of nature and the whole universe … The trip made me lose my boundaries."[62]

The fascinating thing is that all these experiences are characteristic of the consciousness of the ethereal world, including the individual's own ethereal body in that world. Rudolf Steiner describes this as follows in his meditations on achieving a true representation of the ethereal body: "The soul feels the physical body to be separated from the rest of the world; it perceives this only as belonging to it. Thus it is not outside the body with what is experienced in itself. One feels connected to everything that can be called the outside world. One feels connected to things in the surrounding world, just as one feels the sensory world with the hands… One feels completely intertwined and interwoven with what is known as the world. The effects of this pass perceptibly through one's own essence. There is no sharp boundary between the inner world and the outer world … Nevertheless, part of this outside world belongs more to the self than the rest of the surrounding world, just as the head is considered as an independent part in relation to the hands and feet. The soul calls part of the sensory outside world its body. The soul, which has experiences outside this body, can just as well consider part of this non-sensory outside world as belonging to it. If the individual perceives an area that is accessible to him on the other side of the sensory world, he could say that he has a sensory and not perceptible body. This body … could be described as the ethereal body."[63]

Cosmic experience

The ethereal forces are released. Where do they want to go? They strive to return to their place of origin, the cosmos.

Rudolf Steiner describes how plants constantly assimilate ethereal forces from the cosmos so that they can grow and reproduce. These ethereal forces have a cosmic origin and radiate the earth. However, in man these ethereal forces are individualized from the embryonic stage in the form of the ethereal body, so that what is radiated from the cosmos into plants acts on man from the organs of the human body, such as the liver and lungs. A metamorphosis has taken place with regard to the direction of the force; while it passes from the environment onto plants, it works on man from within, from the ethereal body which belongs to him.

As Walther Bühler explained,[64] the ethereal body has a tendency to float away in every direction of the cosmos and dissolve in the distance; the ethereal forces strive to return to their place of origin. However, during a person's life they are prevented from doing so by being connected to the physical body, which is a person's own piece of earth, his or her own substance. In other words, the ethereal forces are bound down. What happens when they are released by the use of LSD?

In this case they have a tendency to float away from us into the surrounding world away from the earth and into space, up to the blue dome of heaven, and as far as the firmament, back to their place of origin. On this voyage, on this trip, they take the user's astral body and self along, and the user reaches a state of ecstasy outside herself, in a weightless world, full of light. Van Ree described this as follows: "The trip made me lose my boundaries and become one with the universe."[62] Others explained: "Suddenly I burst into a vast, new, indescribably wonderful universe."[65] "This trance was like travelling in space, not the external, but the inner person."[77] And finally: "It is kicks, man. It is The Kick. You freak out and there is nothing but greatness and madness. ... If you want to see the galaxies, it's all there."[78]

Again there is a great similarity with the experiences of people who almost died. As Raymond Moody described: "Some people who have had a near-death experience talk about a feeling of floating, quickly rising up into the air so that they see the universe from a perspective which is seen only by satellites and astronauts. The psychotherapist, C.G. Jung, experienced this when he had a heart attack in 1944. He said that he felt that he rose up quickly to a point far above the earth. A child also described the feeling of going up high above the earth, past the stars, finally joining the angels. Another child described how he shot up at great speed and saw all the planets around him, and the earth below looking like a blue marble."[67]

Moody also described how this extraterrestrial world, seen by people who have nearly died, is full of light; they meet creatures made of light. "These creatures do not consist of ordinary light. They shine with such a beautiful intense glow that it looks as though they are penetrating everywhere and are filling man with love. There was even someone who experienced this and said: 'I could describe it as "light" or as "love" and it would come down to exactly the same thing'. Some say that it is almost as though you are flooded by a torrent of light. In addition, they describe the light as being much brighter than any light on earth. And yet, despite its brilliant intensity, it does not hurt the eyes. On the contrary, it is warm, it moves, and it is alive."[68]

This compares with the LSD experience: "Suddenly there was white light and the shimmering beauty of unity. There was light everywhere ... My awareness was acute and complete. ... I felt myself flowing into the cosmos, levitated beyond all restraint, liberated to swim in the blissful radiance of the heavenly visions."[58]

To summarize, we could say that LSD results in the partial death of the user, i.e. part of her ethereal body leaves the physical body, and the ethereal body then dissolves in the world around, becoming one with it. In this context the environment should be seen in very broad terms, reaching from the immediate surrounding area to extra-terrestrial space and up to the firmament. The ethereal forces float back to their place of origin. On their travels, on their trip, they take along the user's astral body and herself, which are joined to it, so that she has a dreamlike experience while remaining awake and conscious of all the impressions which the ethereal body experiences. She sees inner light and sometimes encounters other beings. The light appears to be the perception of the quality of ethereal light which permeates the cosmos and the user's own ethereal body. The creatures which are seen may often be imaginary or a hallucination of individually coloured desires, wishes, fears and so on. However, this is by no means certain. The Huichiol Indians in Mexico used the peyote cactus in their rituals. The most important agent in this cactus is mescaline, which has very similar effects to LSD. It was used, as Van Epen describes, "to achieve a state of ecstasy accompanied by lively, colourful visual hallucinations and visions in which they believed they could communicate directly with the gods."[69]

Therefore it is difficult to have a clear understanding of this area, particularly as the ethereal forces released from the organs of the physical body, and the ethereal forces of the user already dissolved in the surrounding world and in the cosmos, together form an ethereal confusion, with the result that the hallucinations produced from the organs can be combined with the impressions which the ethereal body receives in the (cosmic) outside world. In this case the "inner world" and the "outer world" are confused, and it is not clear what is what.

This brings us to the question whether the LSD user can trust her experiences. Are they a source of extrasensory knowledge, as many users believe, or is this not the case?

The distorting mirror

It is striking that the descriptions of many LSD users refer to grandiose, all-encompassing sights experienced during the LSD trip. However, these insights cannot be "grasped", expressed or passed on. For example, one user wrote: " Soon whole series of thoughts appeared between every word. I had discovered the only true, perfect and original language as spoken by Adam and Eve, but when I tried to explain it, the words I used had little to do with my thoughts. I lost it; that wonderful, valuable, true gift which I should have kept for future generations slipped through my fingers. I felt terrible, and in the end I was no longer able to talk and slipped to the floor... My mind was full of age-old wisdom and I lacked the words to relate it."[70]

There are countless descriptions of this sort. Van Epen characterized them as follows: "Confusion of thought also arises when there is more extensive intoxication (poisoning). For an objective outsider who tries to talk to someone who has taken LSD, it seems as though logic has completely disappeared from his train of thought. The user makes all sorts of associations which do not occur in normal thought. Thus he may make a confused impression, although the capacity for clear and logical reasoning is completely retained by other people who take LSD."[53]

Thus a great deal of confusion is possible; this is easy to imagine because the LSD user is not in any way prepared for the experiences which assail her. She has not had a thorough inner training in which she has learned to develop an understanding of what she observes in the ethereal world outside the physical body. She is unable to "grasp" these experiences, and cannot find the words for them. Nor can she make a clear distinction between the hallucinations produced by the body and the observations of the ethereal world which come to her from the world around her; everything is confused. To make all this even more difficult, the ethereal bodies of other LSD users can also intermingle with her own ethereal body. In this case, all the partly separated ethereal bodies dissolve together and intermingle, becoming one with each other and with the ethereal world around them. Although this process of unification is a blissful one of wordless communication and religious unity, it also creates a great deal of confusion and incomprehension about what is happening. This is the reason that, at the start of the LSD era, many users looked for "travel guides" which describe the life of the soul after death – at least, as it was thousand of years ago – such as *The Tibetan Book of the Dead* and *the Egyptian Book of the Dead*. This also shows that LSD takes the user to the realms of death, because this is where she feels at home and where she feels an urgent need for guidance and help. It was hoped that the above-mentioned ancient books of the dead would provide this.

However, we will return to the question of whether a person who uses LSD can trust her experiences. Are they a source of extrasensory knowledge, or is this not the case?

In the first instance, we can say that when a person uses LSD she surrenders herself for the duration of the trip to a wide range of often chaotically intermingled perceptions, thoughts, feelings, hallucinations etc. which overwhelm her. She will barely be able to distinguish the cause, the relationship and the reality of these. Therefore these experiences do not appear to be a very reliable foundation of knowledge.

And there are other things which are extremely important in this context, and which are fundamental with regard to the reliability and reality of LSD experiences in general. The physical body, which takes up space – volume – is a spatial organism. The ethereal body, which penetrates the physical body and is responsible for all the processes of growth, reproduction, the creation of form, regeneration etc. i.e. for all the life processes which take place in time, is a temporal organism. In order to achieve a healthy and accurate sense of time and space, it is necessary for the physical body and the ethereal body to be correctly linked, so that these two parts fit together exactly and the physical body is completely permeated by the ethereal body. When a person uses LSD, the drug pulls the physical body and the ethereal body apart, with the inevitable result that the user loses a healthy sense of time and space.

Albert Hofmann experienced this, as previously mentioned, during his first deliberate LSD trip: "I also had the feeling that I was not moving forward on my bicycle, though my assistant subsequently told me that we had cycled very fast."

With regard to these experiences, Van Epen wrote: "*Time and space*: the disorientation with regard to time and space deserve to be mentioned. A simple allotment can be experienced like a park in Versailles. A living room with some paintings on the wall can appear to be an art gallery, and a rather chilly, unpleasant room can very easily assume the qualities of a terrible medieval dungeon, filling the tripper with great fear...

"Strange things happen to time, usually in the sense that time is experienced as moving very slowly. Everything that happens seems to take forever. Nevertheless, people still appear to be able to estimate the time fairly accurately while they are under the influence of the drug.

"In a more severe case of LSD poisoning, the sense of time standing still is fairly common, resulting in feelings of infinity and eternity. These feelings can make the user think that she has stepped 'outside time' and finds herself in a sort of 'afterlife'. This can lead to religious and mystical perceptions."[53]

How can these far-reaching changes in the experience of time and space be explained?

In the first place, as regards the experience of time, it is easy to imagine that the user has a feeling of becoming unified with pure time, and that she is living in "infinite" time in a sort of eternity, because her ethereal body, as a temporal organism, is partly dissolved in the ethereal world, i.e. in the world of time, or in a "sea of time".

Secondly, the following factor is very important as regards the experience of time and space. In *The Science of the Secrets of the Soul*, Rudolf Steiner explains that if the human Self and the astral body are not only to be filled with passions and suffering and so on, but are also to be capable of consciously perceiving these, the astral body must be connected with the physical and ethereal body.[71] This is understandable, because when the astral body withdraws from the physical and ethereal body during sleep, this leads to a state of complete unconsciousness, i.e. of deep and dreamless sleep. We will deal with this in greater detail with the description of the effect of marijuana/hashish, but we can say now that in order to have real perceptions, realizations, thoughts, feelings and impulses, it is necessary that these contents of the astral body are reflected by the physical and ethereal bodies which are properly interconnected. When LSD is taken, conscious perceptions, memories, images and so on are experienced as described in detail above, but these contents of the astral body are now reflected in a physical and ethereal body which are not properly connected, so that they cannot be reflected in the correct dimensions of time and space. To repeat Albert Hofmann's words again: "Everything in my field of vision moved back and forth, and was distorted as in a distorting mirror."[11]

Thus the physical and ethereal body reflect the contents of the astral body in a distorted way in terms of size and duration; they do not serve as a mirror, but as a *distorting mirror*. This means that the world experienced by someone who has taken LSD is unreliable. Because of the partial separation of the ethereal body from the physical body, the user sees herself and the world through a mirror which is to some extent a confusing, distorting mirror, and which cannot be trusted. Therefore LSD does not seem to be a reliable source of knowledge, either about oneself (including one's feelings and memories), or of the world, or of the cosmos. It is not, however, completely unreliable because, despite everything, particularly in the case of slight poisoning, there can be a fairly accurate general sense of time and space. In that case only a relatively small part of the ethereal body has become separated, so that there is still a connection with the physical body, allowing for a more or less reasonable reflection of the content of consciousness in time and space. (This also explains Van Epen's experience that, particularly in the case of slight LSD poisoning, it is possible for some people to retain a sense of time and the ability to think clearly and logically. In this case, the reflection is correct in some places.) However, in general it is possible to conclude that the inner and outer world experienced by someone who has taken LSD is usually distorted. Therefore she cannot trust her external perceptions; if she thinks she is able to float or fly from the tenth floor of a building into the clouds, to accompany her departing ethereal body – because she feels at one with the clouds and the ground looks so near – she will actually plummet to the ground. And if she thinks that she can cross the road while a car is hurtling towards her only five metres away, though she believes that it is two hundred metres away, it will be the end of her.

Therefore whatever experiences she has, whether they are sensory perceptions, feelings of leaving the physical body behind, images from a distant past, hallucinations, synaesthesia or the sense of being at one with the world around, these are all reflected onto the senses of a physical body and ethereal body which are not properly inter-connected, i.e. in a sort of distorting mirror, and the user cannot rely on them.

The bad trip

The unreliable and unpredictable character of sensory impressions described above – as well as their possible grotesque distortions, the hallucinations and all the other unexpected experiences, feelings, and so on – can overwhelm an LSD user against her will so that she is at their mercy. This can obviously be very threatening and frightening. Albert Hofmann had his share of this when his sur-roundings changed in a terrifying way as described earlier in this chapter. The woman next door turned into a malevolent and evil witch, and a demon which triumphed over his will entered him mockingly. He wrote: "I was gripped by a terrible fear of going mad. I found myself in another world, in other places with a different time. My body seemed to have no feelings and was lifeless and strange. Was I dying? ... My fear and despair just increased ... My desperate condition ..., the feeling that my physical body was in mortal danger ... a terrible, strange world ... the horrors ...[11] It is clear that an LSD experience can become a horrifying experience full of panic. This is understandable, because the boundary which normally lies between the sensory world and the ethereal world, which protects the unpre-pared person against the overwhelming impressions from this ethe-real world, is violently broken down by the effects of LSD. Therefore Rudolf Steiner warned against the dangers which are incurred by anyone who enters the extrasensory world without the necessary preparation and self-knowledge, because she may be "overwhelmed by the experiences of this world. These experiences can penetrate physical/sensory consciousness in the form of illusions and images. They assume the character of sensory perceptions, with the result that the soul perceives them as being real. But they are not."[72]

They are illusions – resulting from the connection of the ethereal forces dissolved in the ethereal world with the senses of the physical body – and these images and hallucinations, which are, moreover, inaccurately reflected in time and space, can lead to the most violent feelings of fear and panic when LSD is taken. We have encountered a number of examples of this, for example, the person who was horrified when he felt himself, as a flower, being devoured by a strange crawling, terrible black thing, or when he experienced that a huge, slimy snake, a terrible, evil thing, coiled itself around him and swallowed him up. These were all illusions, but the images were present in the process in which part of the ethereal body dissolved in the ethereal outside world. Without the profound self-knowledge which is absolutely necessary (including a knowledge of the individual's own ethereal body, the ethereal world, and of other laws, contents, forces and relationships of other parts of the person as a whole), these images could result in the LSD psychosis described above, i.e. in a paranoid hallucinatory form of schizophrenia which may or may not be long-term.

We will conclude with a final example: "Suddenly I saw an enormous snake. I was scared to death. Another snake appeared and crawled over me. My god! Where did these snakes come from? There appeared to be something behind my back as well. So I looked round and saw a snake which was just about to completely swallow me up. It had arms and legs and a long tail. The end of the tail was like a spear. Oh God, I thought I would surely die. Then I looked the other way and I saw a man with horns and long nails, holding a spear in his hand. He jumped at me like a wild man, and I threw myself to the ground. He missed me. Then I looked around again. He took another run at me and seemed to be aiming his spear at me. Again I threw myself on the ground. There seemed to be no escape ..."[73]

Waking dreams

The next question relates to the consciousness of the LSD user. How do we describe the nature of her consciousness when she has taken the drug?

The first characteristic is that all her perceptions follow each other in an unpredictable way: "I turned into an angel who flew gracefully through space ... Every cell in my body is seething with joyful vibrations. I became a Chinese coolie ..., a fat Turkish sultan ..., silkworms, a cobra. I turned into a huge flash of lightning which cut off the beautiful objects in heaven with a scream."[74] Stanislav Grof, who made a thorough study of the psychological effects of LSD, concluded that there is no single constant symptom, either when he compared different users, or when he compared the various different LSD experiences of one person. Following an analysis of the contents of these experiences, he wrote: "On the basis of more than 3,800 accounts of LSD sessions, I could not isolate a single symptom that was a constant component in every session, and could consequently be considered as a truly unchanging factor."[75] Thus the user is overwhelmed by a huge range and inconceivable deluge of experiences; no matter how much she prepares for taking LSD, she can never know in advance exactly what will happen. She may be affected by any of the phenomena described above, but it is impossible to predict which ones; how; to what degree; in what order; for how long; and with what intensity they will occur.

The second characteristic is that the user is overwhelmed by all her perceptions. She is flooded by a deluge, and is at the mercy of her experiences. She suffers them, and there is no defence or control possible.

These two qualities, the unpredictability of the experiences and their overwhelming nature, are both characteristic of the consciousness of the LSD user. It is like the unpredictable stream of images which pass before the soul of a person who is dreaming, although there may be particular themes characteristic for the person concerned. The difference is that the user is not dreaming; she is awake and is able to direct her senses at the outside world. Therefore her consciousness can be characterized as an enormously intense dreaming consciousness, though this takes place while she is awake: it is like a waking dream.

Flashback

To conclude my study of LSD, I would like to describe another possible consequence of the use of LSD, i.e. the so-called "flashback". A flashback is a trip which occurs spontaneously; in other words, it is like an echo of one or more LSD experiences (when no LSD has been taken). A flashback can occur at the most unexpected moments when, for one reason or another – e.g. as a result of fatigue, tension, a situation that is similar to one during a previous LSD trip, etc. – the ethereal body again partly separates from the physical body. As a result, it is suddenly possible for another LSD experience to take place. This is not difficult to imagine because, when part of the ethereal body has been violently separated from the physical body as a result of using LSD, this creates breaks in the connection between these two parts of the whole body. Because of these breaks, the connection between the physical body and the ethereal body is less stable, and consequently it sometimes takes only a small thing for the ethereal body to break away from the physical body once again. For some ex-LSD users, this has become a chronic matter; they live in constant fear of flashbacks and of succumbing to an LSD psychosis. There is an example of this in *The Weed and the Flower*, the diary of a fifteen-year-old addicted girl: "11 April. Dear Diary,

I do not want to write this down, because I really want to erase it from my mind for good. But I'm so afraid, and perhaps it would be less awful if I told you. Oh diary, help me please. I'm scared. I'm so scared that my hands are sweating, and I'm shaking like a leaf. It must have been a sort of flash of memory, because I was sitting on my bed making plans for Mum's birthday – just what I would buy for her, and how I could turn it into a surprise – when my mind suddenly became completely confused. I can't explain it very well, but it was as though my mind was rolling back, under its own force, and I couldn't stop it in any way. The room became smoky, and I thought I was in an underground shop. We were standing there reading adverts for secondhand rubbish and for everything you could imagine to do with sex. I started to laugh. I felt wonderful. I was the tallest person in the world and I looked down on everyone, and the whole world was full of strange corners and shadows. Then every-thing suddenly changed into a sort of underground film which was very slow and sluggish with crazy lighting. Naked girls were dancing around and making love to statues. I remember one girl licking a statue with her tongue, and it came to life and took her along into the tall blue grass. I couldn't see very well what was happening, but he was obviously making love to her. I was so full of desire that I wanted to burst wide open and run after them, but then I was standing begging in the street and we were all shouting at the tourists: 'How very nice of you. I hope you have a wonderful orgasm with your dog tonight.' Then I had the feeling that I was being smothered, and I was up in the air in the harsh light of rotating lamps and of beams of light. Everything was turning round and round. I was a falling star, a comet boring its way through the firmament in flames. When I finally came to, I was lying naked on the ground. I still can't believe it. I was just lying on my bed thinking about my mother's birthday and listening to records, and suddenly, wham! Perhaps it wasn't a memory. Perhaps I'm schizophrenic. Isn't that what hap-pens to teenagers when they lose contact with reality? Whatever it is, I'm really confused. I don't even have any control over my mind. The words I wrote down when I was out of it are no more than scribbles and wavy lines, mixed up with a load of nonsense and symbols. What should I do? I need someone to talk to. I'm really desperate. Oh God, please help me, I'm so afraid and cold and alone. I have only you, Diary, you and me, a right pair.

"Later: I've done a few maths problems and even read a few pages. At least I can still read. I learnt a few lines by heart, and my mind seems to be working again. I also did some physical exercises, and I think my body is under control. But I wish there were someone to talk to, someone who knows what's the matter and what's going to happen. But there isn't anyone like that, so I'd better forget it. Forget forget, forget, and don't look back. I'll just go on thinking about Mum's birthday. Perhaps Tim and Alex could take her to the cinema after school, and then I'll prepare a delicious meal for when they come back. I'll just pretend it was a nightmare and forget it. Please God, make me forget it, and don't let it happen again. Please, please, please."[76]

Other psychedelic drugs

We will be fairly brief about other psychedelic drugs, because their effects are basically similar to the effects of LSD, though there are some individual differences, particularly with regard to the strength, nature and duration of the symptoms. They are all toxic substances, some of a purely organic nature, some partly or completely synthetic.

The most important purely organic psychedelic substances are psilocybin mushrooms (Central America), fly agaric (Europe, North America, Siberia, Manchuria), and the peyote cactus (North America and Mexico). The active component of the latter is mescaline, which can also be manufactured in a purely synthetic way. An active dose requires approximately 1000 times as much as a dosage of LSD. Some psychedelic substances with a chemical composition include STP, DMT, PCP (Angel Dust), mescaline and MDA.

By no means all these psychedelic substances have the wide range of powerful effects of LSD. For detailed information on these drugs, see J.H. Van Epen's book, *De drugs van de wereld, de wereld van de drugs* (Drugs of the world, the world of drugs), and the above-mentioned, beautifully illustrated book on hallucinogenic plants of the world, written by Albert Hofmann together with Richard Shultes: *Pflanzen der Götter, die magischen Kräfte fer Rauch- und Giftgewächse* (Plants of the Gods, the magic powers of hallucinogenic and toxic plants).

Of the purely organic psychedelic substances, peyote and psilocybin have an effect which is virtually the same as the effect of LSD.

5

Marijuana/hashish

Marijuana and hashish come from the female plant of an annual, *Cannabis sativa* (hemp), which grows wild in large parts of the world. An annual plant is one in which the whole cycle of germination, the development of the leaves, flowering and the formation of the fruit and seeds all take place in one year (from spring to autumn). The male plants have been used for centuries, and the fibres of the stems used to produce paper, thread, canvas and, above all, rope; the female plants produce hemp seed (very popular with birds), as well as marijuana and hashish, which have been very important to many people since ancient times because of their medicinal and consciousness-changing qualities.

The cannabis plant is tall and luxuriant. Depending on the soil conditions and the climate, it can grow from 1 to 5.5 metres tall; the thick hollow stem has many side shoots which have composite leaves, i.e. leaves which all consist of an uneven number of lanceolate, slightly serrated leaflets, spread out in the shape of a fan. All the leaves of the plant are covered with small hairs which secrete a sticky resinous substance. This is distributed over the leaf stems, leaves and bracts, forming a layer of resin which protects the plant against drying out. The higher the leaves are up the plant, the more resin they secrete. The production of resin reaches a peak when the female plants flower: the tops, flowers and leaves are heavy and sticky with resin.

Marijuana and hashish are produced from this resin. It contains toxic substances which can change human consciousness, including tetrahydrocannabinols (abbreviated as THCs), which are the most active in causing changes in consciousness.[1] However, other ingredients of the resin also contribute to this consciousness changing effect, such as, for example, an acid which has an anaesthetizing effect.[2]

Marijuana is no more than the dried and powdered *plant*; the best sort consists of the tops of the flowering female plants, which contain

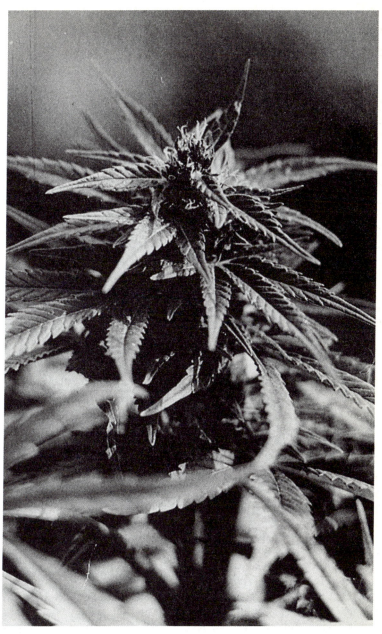

Photograph: The top of a female hemp plant.

a great deal of resin.[3] *Hashish* is the actual *resin*, which can be collected in various ways. One of the methods used is the following: "When the harvested plant is dry enough, the resin turns to powder. This powder can then be shaken off over a cloth or it can be obtained by rubbing the tops between two cloths. The process is repeated a few times, but the dust (resin) which is produced the first time is the best quality. Any leaves and seeds which come off are removed, and the powder is then sieved to remove any smaller extraneous substances (sand). The powder sticks together when it is compressed and is then packaged in bags, kneaded into little balls, or pressed to form blocks. A self-respecting dealer would also emboss a stamp on the blocks as a trademark."[4]

Fairly pure resin (hashish) can be obtained in this way. O'Shaughnessey described a method for producing an even purer form of hashish. He observed the harvest in India in the first half of the nineteenth century: "During the hot season men dressed in leather walked or ran through the fields of hemp, making sure they touched the plants as much as possible. After walking or sprinting through the fields, the resin which stuck to the leather was scraped off with knives and rolled to form balls."[5] A very pure form of hashish is obtained in this way.

Thus there are different techniques for producing hashish; depending on local customs, soil conditions and climate. The well-known types of hashish produced today vary from "Green Turkish", "Red Leb", "Black Afghani", "dark brown Pakistani", and so on. They can vary greatly in purity, and therefore in the content of THC (as a collective name for the tetrahydrocannabinols). In consignments of hashish imported from the Lebanon, Pakistan and India in 1982, the THC content varied from less than 1% to 8%.[6] In general, marijuana ("Congo Grass", "Kenya Grass", "Indian Bhang" etc.) contained between 0.5% and 5% THC. According to the Dutch Central Investigation and Information Department (CRI), the THC content of foreign marijuana/hashish ranged from 0.5 to 14% in 1992."[7]

The more heat and sun the hemp plant gets, the more resin it secretes. In hot, dry areas the resin is secreted abundantly from the swollen, burst glandular sacs protecting the plant from drying out. In cooler, more temperate regions with less sunshine and more rain, the plant produces considerably less resin, and it is therefore of greater interest for supplying strong fibres and seeds than as a source of marijuana and hashish. However, sunshine and heat determine not only the amount of resin that is secreted, but also the concentration of THC in this resin. In more temperate regions (such as the Netherlands) the concentration of THC in the already reduced amount of resin is much lower than in hot, dry regions. Plants grown in artificial conditions however – for example, in well-heated, illuminated greenhouses, living rooms and so on – can have a THC content as high as 10–15% (according to the Netherlands Institute for Alcohol and Drugs), or even 27% (according to the CRI).[7] The consumer can obtain the best quality hashish when the abundant black and very sticky resin is prepared and sold in its pure form, i.e. not mixed with other parts of the plant. In most cases he will smoke it, either on its own or combined with tobacco; it is also possible to eat hashish either in pure form or, for example, cooked in a cake, or to crumble the hashish in drinks.

In the west, marijuana is virtually always smoked, sometimes combined with tobacco, but it can also be chewed or brewed as tea, as is common in India.

A study of the United Nations (in 1950) estimated the number of consumers of marijuana and hashish at more than 200 million people, particularly in Asia and Africa. In comparison with this, the estimated number of alcoholics is over 20 million people, while the number of people who consume alcohol but are not addicted, is about 1 billion. As there has been an enormous increase in the use of marijuana and hashish in the west since 1950, it must be assumed that this drug is one of the most commonly used consciousness-changing substances in the world. The question arises as to why this is the case. What part have marijuana and hashish played in the history of humankind?

Marijuana and hashish in history

The origin of the cannabis plant, one of the oldest plants cultivated by man, probably lies in the highlands of Central Asia. From there the plant spread to *China*, where hemp fibre has been found dating back to approximately 4000 BC. Cannabis is first mentioned in literature in 2737 BC, when the Chinese emperor Shen Nung recommended the plant as a cure for all sorts of ailments, including beri-beri, malaria, constipation, period pains, rheumatic pains, gout, and absent-mindedness (!) In the "Atar Veda" (20th – 14th century BC) the plant is also described as a "source of joy and happiness", and as a "bringer of laughter". However, its use as a means of changing consciousness and contacting the non-visible world took place only on a limited scale in China and, when it was used for this purpose, this was under the guidance of a shaman. For example, in the 5th century BC a Taoist priest described the use of cannabis in combination with ginseng by "people who summon up spirits to speed up time and reveal future events."[8] However, cannabis did not become popular as a means of changing consciousness. In texts dating from roughly the same period, the character for cannabis ("MA") was given a negative accent, referring to its intoxicating properties. It was even given the name "liberator ('loosener') of sin" and subsequently the drug gradually disappeared from Chinese culture. When the first Europeans visited China in approximately 1000 AD, they no longer found cannabis being used as a consciousness-changing drug.

From Central Asia hemp spread in another direction to the west. The warrior knights, the Skythes, introduced hemp in Persia and Mesopotamia from 1500 BC. From there, Persian tribes took seeds of the plants with them on their trips to *India*. This is how hemp reached the Indian culture, where it was believed that the plant had been sent from the world of the gods in order to induce spiritual ecstasy in humankind so that they could contact this world, and in order to instill courage and strong sexual desire. There is a tradition which states: "When the nectar of the Gods dripped from heaven, cannabis sprang up from it."[9] Another tradition relates that "with the help of demons, the gods churned the ocean of milk to prepare nectar for the gods. One of these nectars was cannabis. This was dedicated to Shiva and was Indra's favourite drink. When the ocean had been churned, the demons tried to seize the nectar of the gods, but the gods managed to prevent them. In memory of their victory, they called cannabis 'Vijaya' (victory)."[9] Since then it has been impossible to conceive of the Indian civilization without this gift from the gods; on the one hand, as a medicine, mentioned in the literature in approximately 800 BC, and on the other hand, as a sacred mediator between the gods and humankind.

In Tibet and the Himalayas the plant was also revered; for example, according to a tradition of Mahayana Buddhism, Buddha was supposed to have survived on a single hemp seed per day during the six stages of asceticism which led to his enlightenment (hemp seed is very nutritious and does not have any consciousness-changing properties).

There was a great respect for cannabis throughout India. Bhang (spiced marijuana) was so sacred that it was believed to keep evil forces at bay, to bring happiness, and to purify humans of sin. Sacred oaths were sworn over hemp and it was firmly believed that anyone who trod on the leaves of this holy plant would suffer injury or be afflicted by a great tragedy.

In approximately 1000 AD the use of cannabis had become so popular in India that it was part of daily life and of the religious activities of the population. This continued to be the case. For example, in the 18th century, during great celebrations such as the feast of Vishnu, young priestesses were given hashish to consume. In a trance, they saw the face of god and made predictions. The following passage is a description of these feasts: "At the feasts in the honour of the bloodthirsty goddess Kali, victims were given a drink containing hashish. They were then pushed under the gigantic wheels of a chariot carrying a statue of the goddess. In a trance, others threw themselves before the feet of sacred elephants to be trampled underfoot. According to an estimate made in 1806, the number of victims at these festivities amounted to 20,000 people every year."[10]

1894 saw the publication of a report by the "Indian Hemp Drugs Commission", which was more than 3000 pages long. This study was carried out by the English into the possible damage caused by the use of cannabis in India. The report contained an anthology from the Indian literature on hemp. These are some of the quotations: "The hemp plant is sacred for Hindus ... Dreaming about the leaves, the plant or the sap is a good sign ... It cures dysentery and sunstroke, it dissolves mucus, speeds up digestion, stimulates the appetite, frees the tongue of the lisper, sharpens the intellect and provides energy for the body and joy for the spirit. These are useful and necessary purposes for which the Almighty made bhang in his goodness... In a bhang ecstasy the spark of the Eternal in man casts light on the darkness of matter ... Bhang is the bringer of joy, the flight to Heaven, the Heavenly Guide, the Heaven of the poor, the Comforter of sorrow. In Benares, Ujjain and other holy places, yogis, bairagis and sanyassins used bhang so that they could concentrate their thoughts on the Eternal... With the help of bhang, ascetics could survive for days without food and drink. Many Hindu families safely survived the dreadful misery of famines with the help of bhang. Prohibiting or drastically reducing the use of a herb that is as holy and beneficial as hemp would lead to a great deal of suffering and indignation and would provoke a deep-rooted rage in large groups of revered ascetics. It would rob the people of their comfort in days of hardship, and of a cure for disease and of a guardian whose benevolent protection safeguards them against the attacks of evil influences."[11]

This was one impression taken from Indian literature at the end of the 19th century. Thus it is not surprising that the use of cannabis as a medicine and as a drug is still widespread in India today. The Indian government refuses to implement the World Heath Organization's prohibition of marijuana and hashish, though it does control the cultivation and distribution of the drug.

We will now go back to Persia and Mesopotamia in about 1500 BC, because hemp spread not only to India, but also to the west. The Skythes took the plant to Europe, where the classical world was introduced to the use of cannabis. Heroditus (484-424 BC) described the purification ritual which resulted in religious ecstasy during Skythe funerals as follows: "The Skythes take some of this hemp product, and after crawling under canvas (tents), they throw it onto glowing hot stones. It immediately smokes, producing steam which cannot be surpassed by any Greek steam bath. The Skythes then cheer jubilantly (because they inhale the smoke), and for them this steam takes the place of bathing in water, because they never ever wash the body with water." (12) He also described a people who lived by the River Araxes, who threw the herb in the fire and inhaled the smoke during their religious ceremonies. According to Heroditus, inhaling this smoke "made them just as drunk as the Greeks become when they drink wine". (13) Thus the *Greek* and later also the *Roman* civilization – which used hemp predominantly for making rope, canvas and clothes – were familiar with the con- sciousness- changing properties of the plant. Democritus wrote that on special occasions cannabis was drunk together with wine and myrrh in order to summon up visions; in Thebes, an opium-like drink was prepared from hemp, and in approximately 200 AD Galen described how hemp was sometimes used in a sweet dessert, which was eaten together with a sweet drink, to put the guests into a merry mood after the meal. It is not possible to say with any certainty whether cannabis was used as a drug in the Mysteries and Oracles. However, in 1975, many blocks of hashish were discovered under- neath the ruins of the Oracles of the Dead in Ephira in northern Greece. Chapter 2 described how drugs played an extremely impor- tant role in the Oracles and during the initiation process of the Mysteries, but the question of whether marijuana and hashish were used for this remains unanswered.

In the burgeoning *Arab* culture the use of marijuana and hashish was increasingly integrated. For example, the joys of hashish were praised in many writings in Arab literature, such as the "Tales of the Thousand and One Nights", which were permeated with the sweet smell of hashish. However, abuse of the drug was widespread. In about the 8th century AD, the use of hashish was prohibited in Egypt and severe penalties were imposed. In the 10th century, measures were also introduced in many other places to prevent excessive use of the drug.

Roughly after the First Crusade (1099 AD), hashish also acquired a new aspect. The drug was used by the secret society of the Assassins, founded by Al-Hassan-ibn-al-Saddah (died 1124). Based in his fortress, the Alamut, Hassan had founded a fanatical religious terrorist order which instilled terror in the Christian Crusaders and in the Arab population over a wide area (Palestine, Syria, Iraq, Persia). He had political opponents liquidated to increase his own territory. These murders were committed by "fidawis", who risked their own lives. They were on the bottom rung of the organization, and made the attacks rather like suicide commandos. Marco Polo, who visited the Alamut in 1271 or 1272, described how Hassan managed to get them to do this.

First, he described the paradisical gardens and the elegant pavilions which Hassan had built, and then he continued: "No one had access to the Garden except those who were destined to become Ashishins. At the entrance there was a fortress which was strong enough to repel the whole world, and there was no other way of entering the Garden. There were a number of young men at the Court between the ages of twelve and twenty who had a taste for military exploits. They were allowed to enter the Garden, sometimes in groups of four, six or ten at a time, after they had first drunk a special drink which caused them to fall into a deep sleep (according to tradition, the drink contained strong hashish). Then they were carried into the Garden so that they woke up there. When they woke up and discovered that they were in such charming surroundings, they thought that were in Paradise. There were ladies and girls who frolicked and caressed them to their hearts' desire. When the Old Man (Al-Hassan-ibn-al-Saddah) wished to have a prince murdered, he would tell one of the youths: 'Go and kill such and such a person; when you return, my angels will transport you to Paradise, and should you die, I will also send my angels to bring you to Paradise.' "[14] The order existed from 1090 to 1257. In that year the Mongols vanquished the kingdom of the Assassins and destroyed the secret society on their victorious march to the west. The descendants of the Assassins were dispersed across northern Syria, Iran, Zanzibar (an island off the coast of Tanzania), and above all, India, where they are known as Thojas and Mowlas; their spiritual leader was called the Seventh Imam, and is known to the rest of the world as the Aga Khan.[14]

The name given by the Crusaders is a reminder of the role played by hashish in the society: they called them "Hashishins" (users of hashish), and this later led to the word Assassins. The murderous character of the order has been retained in the word assassin, or murderer.

Let us return to the Arab world. Despite the various prohibitions and the threat of severe penalties, it proved to be impossible to banish the use of the drug. For many people the consumption of hashish continued to be an important part of daily life. This was also the case in *Egypt*: Martin Schouten wrote that "in 1402 a puritanical reformer ordered all hemp to be removed from the Djoneina Garden, a place of pleasure where ladies enjoyed cultivating hemp and serving hemp products to their clients. In order to enforce the prohibition, it was decreed that any girl who was caught with ganja (the dried flowering tops) would immediately have all her teeth extracted. However, the historian wrote that within a few years its popularity had increased more than ever."[15]

From Egypt the drug spread to the countries of North Africa and to central, eastern and southern *Africa*, where Hottentots, Bushmen, Pygmies, Kaffirs and many other tribes used cannabis as a medicine and intoxicating drug. It also played a role in their cult practices and rituals as a consciousness-changing substance. For example, Hofmann and Schultes described how "the Kasai tribes from Zaire revived an ancient Riamba cult by elevating hemp, rather than the old fetishes and symbols, as a god and protector against physical and spiritual harm. Agreements were sealed with clouds of smoke from waterpipes made of pumpkins."[16]

According to some historians, the practice of the ingestion of hemp was brought to *America* from Africa by negro slaves. Here it fell on fruitful ground because the Spaniards had already introduced the plant there (for the manufacture of rope, canvas, clothes), and had started cultivating hemp, for example, in 1545 in Chile, and in 1554 in Peru. However, according to other researchers, both cannabis and the religious and ritual use of the plant were already in use in America before Columbus. They believed that the Aztecs in Central America and tribes of North American Indians had already used cannabis during their religious ceremonies.

Hemp was first planted by the English in Jamestown (in the *United States*) in 1611 for the shipping industry (to make rope and canvas). The cultivation of hemp later became extremely important for the textile industry, but it was not used in any way as a drug.

However, this changed in the course of the nineteenth century when several doctors, writers and artists, such as Lewis Carroll, John Stuart Mill and William James started to experiment with marijuana and hashish. Its use was restricted to a small group until Mexican immigrant workers imported the drug into the southern United States in the first quarter of the *twentieth century*. In those days marijuana was cheaper than alcohol, and when the use of alcohol was actually prohibited in 1920, the use of marijuana became increasingly attractive to the population groups working with Mexicans, such as negroes, uneducated white labourers, sailors etc. New Orleans became the centre where smoking marijuana was taken over from the Mexicans. According to some alarming newspaper stories, in 1926 the whole city, from the underworld to the social elite, and from the entertainment district to the schools, had "succumbed" to marijuana.[17] The crews of the Mississippi steamboats spread the use of the drug from New Orleans to the midwest and the north of the United States. Marijuana was being smoked in New York by 1921 and, by 1930, there was virtually no city left in the United States where it was not smoked. However, its use remained restricted to the so-called lower social classes (and artistic circles). It was most popular in the black ghettos in the big cities. Jazz music sang the drug's praises: "Muggles" (Louis Armstrong, 1928) "Chant of Weed", Don Redman (1931) "Sweet Marijuana Brown", (Barney Bigard, 1945) "Stoned" (Wardle Gray, 1948). In 1937, the supply and possession of marijuana became virtually impossible as a result of the "Marijuana Tax Act", probably as a result of pressure from the alcohol industry, since alcohol had been legalized again in 1933. Very high taxes were levied on the possession of marijuana: 100 dollars an ounce. Anyone who did not pay was fined a maximum of

2000 dollars and sentenced to five years in prison.

However, despite the forceful national campaigns and the destruction of tons of marijuana, its consumption continued to smoulder during the 1940s and 1950s. It once again became popular with students and the youth movement in the 1960s through jazz music, white artists and intellectuals, and there was an explosive increase in consumption.

In 1965, the American poet Allen Ginsberg wrote: "The most important poets, painters, musicians, film makers, sculptors, actors, singers and publishers in America and England have been smoking marijuana for years. I have been high with most of the poets whose contributions are included in the Don Allen anthology of new American poetry 1945-1960; and, in the years following its publication, I have also had a cup of coffee and smoked a joint with quite a few of the more academic poets of the competing Hall-Pack-Simpson anthology. No exhibition can open now in Paris, London, New York or Wichita without the incense of marijuana wafting out when the door of the ladies' toilet opens".[18] At the end of the 1960s it was estimated that more than one-third of all university students and hundreds of thousands of college and high school students had smoked marijuana and hashish. In addition, countless American soldiers in Vietnam regularly used cannabis. Next to LSD, it was *the* drug of the hippy movement. Consumption assumed epidemic proportions, and during a conference in San Francisco in 1986, reference was even made to an explosive increase in the number of marijuana and hashish *addicts*. These were mainly young people whose parents used cannabis as a so-called "social" drug – i.e. the second generation of marijuana and hashish users.[19]

Finally, to *Europe*. Following its introduction by the Skythes, cannabis did not play a significant role as a consciousness-changing drug until the mid-nineteenth century, though the plant may have been used in various late medieval witches' potions. On the other hand, hemp had been very popular since Graeco-Roman times for its fibres, which were used to make clothes, canvas and rope. It was grown in Gaul from the third century BC, where its fibres were much stronger because of the cooler climate. From there they were transported to countries further south. Cannabis was also mentioned as a medicine, although its dangers were recognized: "Medieval herbalists made a distinction between 'composted' (cultivated) and inferior hemp, and recommended the latter for swellings caused by gout, growths and other hard tumours, and the former as a medicine for a whole series of diseases from coughs to jaundice. However, they warned against using the drug excessively, as this could lead to sterility; in men 'it dried out the seed', in women the 'milk in their breasts'."[20] Medical texts dating from the seventeenth and eighteenth century referred to hemp several times as a useful medicine, although it "fills the head with vapours" (*The New London Dispensatory*, 1682) and as a compound which produces a mood of gaiety (Alexander, 1763). However, there was no sign of widespread use either for medical or non-medical purposes.[21]

All this changed, as it did in the United States, in the course of the nineteenth century, when Napoleon's soldiers probably brought hashish back to France from Egypt. Furthermore, when the doctors, O'Shaughnessy, Aubert-Roche and Moreau de Tours studied its use in India and the United States, and Moreau de Tour wrote his fundamental book (*Du haschisch et de l'Aliénation Mentale*) in 1845, interest in this drug gradually increased. Initially there was great enthusiasm, particularly with regard to the tranquillizing and anaesthetizing qualities of hashish. Later on, cannabis was recommended for many different complaints. In the second half of the nineteenth century, extracts of the drug could be bought in virtually every apothecary. However, Moreau de Tours' study also aroused great interest amongst his artistic and literary friends in Paris. They founded the "Club des Haschischins" and met in the Hotel Pimodan in the Latin Quarter to use the drug. Writers like Charles Baudelaire, Théophile Gautier, Arthur Rimbaud and Gérard de Nerval later described their experiences, and Baudelaire's *Les paradis artificiels* has become particularly famous. However, its use remained restricted to this artistic circle.

Until the Second World War, there was virtually no significant consumption of marijuana and hashish in Europe except in Southern Russia and Greece. In southern Russia, in about 1930, the drug was imported from Asia Minor. In Greece, it was used quite a lot around the First World War because of the extensive cultivation of hemp, until this was prohibited in 1920 and this prohibition was actually implemented in 1936. Later, cannabis became established because immigrants, from countries where the use of marijuana and hashish was part of the cultural pattern for many people, brought their customs with them to Europe: Jamaicans and Africans to England, immigrants from Surinam to the Netherlands, North Africans to France. Apart from these groups, the interest was restricted to jazz musicians, who came into contact with it through their American colleagues, and to artists who adopted its use. It was not until the late 1950s that the use also became widespread amongst young people, and in the course of the 1960s there was an explosive rise in consumption in Europe, as there was in the United States. Hippies, students, secondary schoolchildren, young working people and other, mostly young, people incorporated the consumption of cannabis into their lifestyles, initially as a substance for expanding consciousness and, later, increasingly merely for pleasure, or as a remedy for inner restlessness, loneliness and emptiness.

Here are some of the figures: the quantity of cannabis seized in West Germany in 1968 was 380 kilos. In 1979, it was 6,407 kilos, and in 1987, more than 11,000 kilos. In the Netherlands (the centre of the trade) it was 2,315 kilos in 1972, 17,919 kilos in 1979, 68,238 kilos in 1988, 109,752 kilos in 1990, and 96,292 kilos in 1991.[a] (In Germany it is assumed that the quantity of illegally traded cannabis is approximately ten times the amount that is seized.) In the Netherlands the number of people who used cannabis in 1988 was estimated at half a million. The drug is sold in coffee shops, discotheques, youth centres etc. Anyone who is looking for cannabis can find it without any problem, and use it without fear of punishment.

To summarize, it may be said that the use of marijuana and hashish, which has continued in Asia, Africa, the Arab world and in South and Central America up to the present day, has risen to record heights because of the explosive increase in consumption in the western world. Cannabis is undoubtedly the most widely used hallucinogenic drug in the world. In the west, this drug from the east has become part of the arsenal of consciousness-changing substances available to young people. For example, in the United States the percentages of eighteen-year-olds who had used cannabis were 47% in 1975, 60% in 1980, and 50% in 1987.[22] In the Netherlands these percentages were 16% in 1975, 15.5% in 1980, and 18% in 1987.[22,b] A study published in 1987 showed that 4% of American eighteen-year-olds had used cannabis twenty times or more in the preceding month. In the Netherlands this percentage was found to be 3.1% of seventeen- to eighteen-year-old pupils in Amsterdam.[22] According to the Dutch Information Service for Alcohol and Drugs, the number of cannabis users registered for treatment has increased in recent years, particularly amongst young people.

The effects of marijuana and hashish

It is by no means simple to describe the effects of marijuana and hashish on the various aspects of the human organism, because cannabis has such an extensive range of possible effects. On the one hand, it has hallucinogenic properties, but on the other, it has anaesthetizing effects which produce a dreamy, sleepy mood. It can also – especially in the form of marijuana – be used as a light stimulant. Because these effects can alternate and overlap during the use of the drug, it is difficult to predict exactly what the effects of marijuana and hashish will be. However, there is a difference between the various sorts of cannabis with regard to the particular effect which is emphasized. For example, Kif (the dried resin and tops of the North African plant) generally has a more stimulating effect, while for many people, Afghani and Nepalese hashish produce a more passive mood, with hallucinogenic effects. There is also the different THC content of various cannabis products, which in turn contributes to the diverse intensity of experiences. Thus within the range of effects described here, the drug is able to produce different effects on the user in terms of the nature and intensity of the experience. Therefore a regular user will try to buy the type and quality of cannabis which produces the effects that suit him best. One person will prefer Red Leb, another Black Afghani, and yet another will opt for Kif, etc. Despite these differences with regard to the specific effects, we will endeavour to present a comprehensive picture of the influence which cannabis has on the different aspects of the human organism.

To do this it is necessary to know what happens to the active components of cannabis (particularly THC) in the human body. Numerous scientific studies on humans and animals, including studies with traceable radioactive THC, reveal that despite individual differences, these active components go into the brain. For example, one hour after giving monkeys the radioactive THC, high concentrations were found particular in the cortex, and in the deeper parts of the brain, the so-called basal ganglia.[23] These basal ganglia include, amongst other things, the centres which are related to the experience of feelings such as pleasure, discomfort, and so on.

In addition, the active components of cannabis reach the rhythmic system of the human organism, i.e. those parts which are in continuous rhythmic motion such as, in particular, the lungs (respiration) and the heart (circulation of the blood). This is easy to imagine, because the toxins in marijuana and hashish, which are virtually always smoked, in the first instance enter the lungs; from there they make their way to the heart and the circulation, to be distributed round the whole body. In the lungs, THC causes a widening of the bronchia,[24] and in the heart and circulation it initially leads to an increase in heartbeat by almost one-third, which is dangerous for anyone with a heart condition. In addition, the blood vessels in the whites of the eyes dilate, giving the user red, bloodshot eyes (rabbit's eyes). Furthermore, the peripheral blood vessels are constricted, resulting in cold hands, feet, ears and the tip of the nose. As THC reaches the glandular and lymph systems, it inhibits the functioning of the salivary muscles, resulting in a dry throat and mouth.

In addition, the active components of cannabis reach the whole of the rest of the body, because THC has the property, like DDT, of adhering to the fatty tissues and consequently it is excreted extremely slowly.[25] Thus tests on animals showed that only 17-40% of the radioactive THC had been expelled from the body within 24 hours, and that after a week more than 50% of the original dose was still in the body in the form of metabolic traces (waste products).[26] An experiment with volunteers showed that eight days after being given a single dose of radioactive THC (injected into the blood) 20-30% remained in the body in the form of metabolic traces[27]; even thirty days after being taken, chemical traces of THC could still be found.[28]

Summarizing the findings mentioned above, it is clear that far-reaching changes are caused by cannabis in all these areas – in the (fatty) brain tissue, in the rhythmic system and in the other fatty tissues of the human body, including the digestive organs and the limbs – i.e. in the body as a whole. This is very different from LSD, which, like mescaline, has a much more limited scope of operation. It hardly enters the brain and goes virtually only to the kidneys and liver. However, marijuana/hashish has a much wider area of operation and spreads through the whole body, influencing it almost everywhere.

What is the effect of marijuana/hashish on the different aspects of the human organism? We will try to explain this by describing the course of a cannabis "high".

The course of a marijuana/hashish "high"

Looking at the course of a marijuana/hashish "high" reveals that, when it is smoked, the experience lasts from two to four hours and, allowing for individual differences and the strength of the dose, broadly speaking has the following pattern.

It often starts with a perception of all the earthly realities in relative terms. This applies to normal perceptions and the ideas related to them – details can suddenly become much more important – and to patterns of habits, arrangements, time duration, spatial distances etc. They all become much more relative, different and amusing. It is as though one is removed from them. Here is an example from Martin Schouten's book, *Marijuana and Hashish*: "It starts when you're standing in front of an open wardrobe getting undressed and ready to go to bed. You have to fall asleep quickly, because you have to get up in four hours' time to check the stove, which isn't working very well. However, it is even more important to get a contract to the office as quickly as possible. Mike telephoned to say that he had finished the investment plan, and it's high time to phone George. You feel tense. You are high and you know it. But then you think about it a bit and tell yourself that there's no reason to hurry to go to sleep. It's completely crazy! Hurry to go to sleep? All these things occur to you as you are taking off a sock, and suddenly you relax. Time isn't all that important after all, and surely you're the master of your own time. No one else is. You say to yourself: 'Good heavens, am I really in such a rush?' Is time that important? You decide to enjoy taking off your other sock, and you think that no one should be in such a hurry. It just means you're one step nearer your grave, and it's good fun taking off a shirt."[29]

When the mood described above is even stronger, and there is a great deal of laughter while the marijuana and hashish "high" is developing, this can lead to the giggles. Van Epen describes that "even when there is no suggestion of a funny situation, users can burst out laughing. Their laughter is contagious for other users, but outsiders are often rather surprised by the silly giggling."[30]

A study of the effects mentioned so far, particularly of the spontaneous laughter, shows that there is a partial separation of the astral body from the ethereal and physical body. The laughter is actually an expression of the fact that the astral body momentarily withdraws from the ethereal and the physical bodies, so that the astral body can expand elastically in the surrounding space and is largely liberated from them for a while. Rudolf Steiner discusses this as follows: "When a person rises up above himself, the astral body expands like an elastic substance and becomes slack, though it is usually tense.

When the astral body expands, it liberates the person from the bond with the other parts of his being; it is as though he is withdrawing into himself and raising himself up above the whole situation. Because everything which happens in the astral body expresses itself in the physical body, this withdrawal is also expressed; the expansion of the astral body into the physical body is expressed in laughter or a smile."[31]

This is what happens to a large extent when a person gets high. The user feels an "upward movement". He gets high and rises up above the situation and above the normal pattern of behaviour of the ethereal body, looking down on it, seeing it in relative terms and laughing uncontrollably about it when he succumbs to the giggles. Things get really out of hand when the user finds that these experiences are combined with the distorted images of reality which appear as though in a distorting mirror, and even with hallucinations.[32] The uncontrolled laughter then reaches a peak.

In short, it is clear that the effects of marijuana and hashish result from the astral body partially separating from or raising itself above the ethereal and physical body. This process, i.e. the expansion, slackening and relaxation of the usually rigid astral body so that it partly floats up and becomes high, produces a liberated, light and relaxed feeling. The physical body remains languid with slack muscles, heavy as a stone – "stoned". The user feels stoned, relaxed, loose and high, and it feels good.

The writer of *The Weed and the Flower* described this: "At last it started to work, just when I thought it would never happen, and I felt myself becoming happy and as free as a bird in the high blue sky. I was so relaxed. I don't think that I've ever felt as relaxed as this in my life. It was wonderful!"[33]

But it can also be different. When part of it has become separated, the astral body can displace its scope of operation elsewhere, and forcibly connects with the organs of the rhythmic system (the heartbeat is faster) and above all with the digestive organs and the muscular system so that, shortly after taking the drug, the user suddenly becomes active, feels restless and even hyperactive. He wants to go into the world and move about; his astral body forces him to do so. This aspect of his being has descended even further into, amongst other things, the musculature of the limbs. The user feels that he has extra strength and power. In this case, cannabis works as a light stimulant, though it does not usually last long. The connections which have been made are unstable and break down after a while, so that the user calms down.

In addition, there may be a number of symptoms at the start of the high, which will be described in more detail, such as changes in the user's train of thought and an intensification of sensory impressions.

What are the phenomena which predominate as the high continues? Although it is impossible to predict the user's experiences exactly – for this depends on his personality and mood, the time when the drug is taken and its quality and strength etc. – it is possible to conclude that the following effects are the most common:
- changes in sensory perception;
- changes in thinking, feeling and the will;
- changes in the sense of time and space;
- an increasing sleepiness and dreaminess.

Changes in sensory perceptions

All sensory perceptions – particularly the senses of sight and hearing, but also the senses of smell, taste and touch – are experienced more profoundly and with great intensity and sensitivity. Sounds become fuller and deeper, colours brighter and more saturated etc.

This is described in *The Weed and the Flower* as follows: "Then I ate a salted peanut and I noticed that I had never before tasted anything as salty. I felt that I was a child again, and was trying to swim in the great salt lake, but the peanut was even saltier than that! My liver, my spleen and my intestines were completely eroded by the salt."[34] However, this does not by any means mean that sensory impressions are perceived more acutely externally. (The perception threshold does not fall.) In fact, the opposite seems to be the case when hallucinogenic substances are taken; it is only inwardly that sounds, colours, tastes etc. are experienced in a richer and fuller way and more intensely and sensitively. They are permeated with greater feeling, with an inner life, a spiritual life. Life and feelings become connected to perceptions. The forces of ethereal light[32] or the forces of light and life, are released by the effect of marijuana/hashish from the sphere of the kidneys and the nervous system and become connected with the ethereal forces of the nervous and sensory system in other places. They connect, in particular, to the senses so that there are more intense, vibrant sensory perceptions in the astral body. They also have a greater feeling content. This reveals that the astral body (the carrier of our feelings of pleasure, suffering, joy, sorrow etc.), which has become partly separated, becomes connected to the sensory processes so that these are experienced with a greater content of feeling. We will return to this aspect below.

Changes in thinking, feeling and the will

As regards *thinking*, it is very striking that when the user takes a fairly large dose of cannabis, he loses the "red thread" of logic and purposeful will in his thinking. His thoughts often flit from one thing to another. He can become confused and chaotic, and his thinking is associative. He can also be overwhelmed by an incessant stream of fantastic ideas which he finds difficult to articulate because they are just too crazy, completely mad. His thoughts lose contact with earthly realities because he starts to make all sorts of associations which do not correspond to reality, and which a non-user can no longer follow. This is certainly related to the fact that, as described above, THC causes changes in the brain which prevent it from adequately performing its task as a mirror for thinking.

What exactly does it mean when we describe the task of the brain as a mirror for thinking? In order to clarify this, we must digress briefly to describe the activity of thinking in terms of spiritual science. We will begin by stating that by thinking we mean the inner activity of thinking, which the self wishes to engage in, and not the unrelated pattern of associated ideas and conditioned images which rise up in the soul more or less of their own accord. True thinking is always directed by the will. This thinking can be seen as an activity that is "free of the body", i.e. as an activity which takes place *in* the soul and *outside* the body and which serves, with the help of the brain, to grasp, perceive and understand the world of concepts. We immediately become conscious of this activity of thinking because this effort is impressed on the physical and ethereal aspects of the brain, leaving traces in them, and reflected by them, with the result that the soul can become aware of these reflections in the form of thoughts and images. In other words, the spiritual activity of thinking which is directed by the will takes place in the soul, outside the body, and the process of this activity is impressed on the physical and ethereal aspects of the brain, which in turn allow this imprint to flower in the soul, where it becomes conscious in the astral body. This seems a long-winded process but, because it follows this path, thinking is an eminently *free* process – it does not have to be disturbed by all sorts of associations and patterns of images which are found in the complex of the physical and ethereal body, and bubble up in consciousness. It should be clear that this perspective contrasts with the usual view that thinking is a function of the physical brain, that it is produced by the brain and that it is a result of the biochemical and electrical processes in the brain. We do not define true thinking in this way, though we do recognize that this applies to random thoughts, images and associations which are forced up from the ethereal body of the brain into consciousness. True thought, in the words of L.F.C. Mees, is "no more a function of the brain than playing the piano is a function of the piano. Someone plays the piano; the piano is the instrument which serves the player. Man needs his brain to think, but he himself is thinking and his brain is merely the instrument for this purpose."[35]

This instrument is influenced by THC. As a result, the brain of someone who uses marijuana or hashish becomes a rather unstable mirror surface, and because of this effect, shreds of ethereal forces can be released in the form of associations and images. In short, seen from the bottom, the potentially clear and tranquil reflecting "sea" becomes restless and chaotic, and therefore less reliable as a mirror.[36]

The question which arises is what happens to the ethereal and astral forces released *from the brain?*

The ethereal forces can lead, on the one hand, to the development of hallucinations and visions (see Chapter 4: LSD) and, on the other hand, they can also expand in the ethereal cosmos and, in the case of a high dose, produce the effects described for LSD trips, or connect with the ethereal forces in other parts of the body. In this case, cannabis intensifies sensory perceptions.[32]

What happens to the astral forces of the head, where the Self is embedded? There is an extremely interesting lecture by Rudolf Steiner which provides an answer to this question. He explains that when a person goes to sleep, the astral body and the Self expand, on the one hand, into the astral and spiritual world, while on the other hand, they become closely connected in the head with the physical and ethereal organism which has fallen asleep. The astral body connects to the nervous system of the spinal cord and the Self becomes connected with the autonomous or vegetative nervous system (which regulates involuntary physical processes, such as respiration, glandular secretions etc.).[37]

This is extremely important because it allows for the question of what happens when this process takes place, at least partially, in the waking state as a result of special circumstances, such as the effects of a drug.

The result is a change in consciousness. According to Steiner,[37] this change in consciousness makes it possible to perceive with the feelings those things which normally remain concealed below the threshold of consciousness, viz.: the wisdom which permeates the whole world and which unifies creation as a whole.

One user described his high as follows: "It is as though each grain of sand, each leaf, is exactly in the right place and is perfectly taken care of and finished off. I feel a tendency to become immersed and concentrate on it fully."[38] In *Marihuana en hasjiesj* (Marijuana and Hashish), Martin Schouten wrote: "There is a force which connects and permeates the world and all its parts, and which the smoker also feels in himself, a context in which he feels incorporated."[38]

In the historical description we encountered the experience described above as one of the traditionally important reasons for using cannabis, particularly in the east: the mystical experience that divine wisdom permeates the whole world, making all creation one. Marijuana and hashish users experience this directly and *feel* this knowledge, which is experienced full of love. It may sound very strange, but Steiner said: "When love develops between two people, the connection between the autonomous nervous system and the Self, and between the astral body and the system of the spinal cord, are unconsciously active in ordinary life to a high degree."[37]

Thus we can also say that, as these connections have been made as a result of the effect of the drug, this leads to a feeling of love for the omnipresent wisdom in the world. It is an eminently mystical experience which takes place, an experience which is new and which cannot, or can hardly be, understood in analytical terms. Often it can only be very clumsily articulated. In other words, because the astral body and the Self have already partly left the brain during the waking state, something happens which normally happens only in sleep, with the result that during a high the user finds himself in a state which is somewhere in between waking and sleeping. He is in a sort of "dream" while he is still awake.

This is an experience which, as described in chapter 2, can be compared with the normal state of consciousness of mankind in very ancient times, when the world of the gods and the world of man were still one, and when the omnipresent divine wisdom was still experienced by everyone as being self-evident, in a sort of dream. This state of consciousness was lost in the course of time; the world of the gods gradually withdrew from consciousness, and man increasingly woke up to the earth and felt alone and abandoned, with an increasing inner desire for this ancient past. Since several thousand years BC, cannabis has been used to satisfy this desire.

In his book, *Soft drugs*, M. Kooyman wrote: "Cannabis has been used in the East since ancient times as a way of achieving a mystical experience in which the divine presence is felt in man and all things. Buddhists use cannabis for a mystical experience which focuses on achieving detachment from earthly things."[39]

Thus we see that the effect of cannabis brings about an ancient state of consciousness, though nowadays this is at the expense of a clear, sober and logical intellect. Part of the astral forces and the forces of the Self have had to leave the brain, and are therefore no longer sufficiently present there to allow concentrated thinking. As described above, the user has in a sense become a dreamer. When he does attempt to think in a purposeful and logical way, he is handicapped because he will have to rely on forming concepts on an out-of-tune instrument damaged by the effect of THC – to use L.F.C. Mees's analogy. In short, it will be difficult for him to have a reliable knowledge and understanding of his experiences.

All these things explain why, for many (young) people, marijuana/hashish has been the substance chosen (in addition to LSD) since the mid-1960s to fulfil their – usually unconscious – inner demand for knowledge and wisdom, love and togetherness. The experiences they had when they were high answered this need, but the price was high: many abandoned western ways of thinking, gave up their studies or left their professions and became so-called "drop outs", leaving the development of western society to others. Although the feelings of love and being at one with the universe, which they experienced when they were high, were communicated to the world ("hippy, flower power, love-ins, make love not war") and they acquired a new "ecological" consciousness, many people no longer joined in the rat race of a society directed towards performance. They saw through the spiritual poverty of high marks, ambitious careers and clinging onto old structures and old ways of thinking. They mocked the poor suckers who continued on that path, and abandoned it themselves. In fact, this resigned attitude suited the establishment at the time very well. For in those turbulent days of student unrest and so on, a satisfied smoker did not rock the boat!

Many people turned to the East for knowledge. Ancient eastern texts and meditation techniques became popular. People rejected western ways of thinking which attempted to explain all phenomena in purely intellectual and materialistic terms, leaving no room for admiration and love of divine creation full of wisdom.

People sought each other, looking for a togetherness which was also helped (and is still helped) by the use of cannabis, in the following way. So far we have mentioned only the part of the astral forces and the forces of the Self which leave the brain to become attached to the nerves of the spinal cord and of the autonomic nervous system respectively. All we said about the other part of the astral forces and forces of the Self which are released is that they leave the brain when a person falls asleep, and expand in the astral and physical world. The experiences of togetherness and of intense contact which users can have when they get high together are explained by this. Part of the users' astral bodies become detached, with the result that all the partially separated astral bodies containing the Self can expand in the astral world, mixing together, fusing together and becoming one. This produces a sense of unification, and an experience of unity and intense contact, which is further reinforced by deep feelings of sympathy and love, that are evoked by the connection of the other part of the astral body and the Self with the nerves of the spinal cord and the autonomic nervous system respectively.

To the outsider this appears to have a rather exclusive character for, as a non-user, he literally stands outside the experience. He does not share the partial process of astral fusion experienced by the users: "They (non-users) are so far removed that you do not have any contact with them." However, as a user, you are in contact with other users, which is why marijuana and hashish are such attractive consciousness-changing drugs, particularly for young people, who often long for feelings of closeness and friendship with their peers when they are adolescents. "Blowing dope" together, they enjoy the sense of togetherness in the astral world!

However, the problem is that this happens during a state of partial astral separation while, in fact, during puberty the astral body actually wishes to enter the body as a whole, so that it can gradually become a suitable instrument for the rest of the adolescent's life.[40] And yet the young smoker actually moves in the opposite direction: he lets his newborn astral body fuse and dissolve, losing its identity in the astral world at a time when the astral body should be developing its own unique structure and form through experience, assimilation and learning to cope with feelings of joy, sadness, sympathy, antipathy, contact, loneliness etc.

Cannabis stops this process taking place. Instead, the partly separated astral body produces the above-mentioned experiences of warm, mystical security, a creation full of wisdom, an intense contact and togetherness in a group of other users and a much more emotional experience of sensory perceptions, images and thoughts. However, it should be remembered that cannabis does not give anything for nothing. It is possible to remain inwardly passive and stay on the sidelines. If it is taken regularly, the user cannot develop personal feelings and emotions based on love and suffering. These remain static, and the possibilities of adolescence are "dreamed away". That is why people who have regularly smoked cannabis – for example, those who started at fourteen and have smoked marijuana and hashish almost daily for ten years, are obviously physically older than fourteen by the time they are twenty-four, though they still have many of the psychological characteristics of early adolescence. When they stop using the drug, they still have a large part of puberty and adolescence to go through.

Thus feelings are strengthened by the effect of marijuana and hashish. In *Soft Drugs*, M. Kooyman wrote: "Existing feelings are intensified by the use of the drug."[41] He added: "For example, pain, fear, suspicion and melancholy can become more intense."[41] This is the other side of the coin; when the burden of feelings of melancholy and insecurity, which already weigh upon the soul, are strengthened by the additional astral forces released, to such an extent that these feelings lead to an overwhelming mood of depression and fear.

In addition, as a result of the partial separation of the ethereal body from the physical body caused by the toxin THC, there may also be phenomena such as those described for LSD – or at least some of them. They include the processes of partial death as expressed in the release of emotions and memories, of frequently intensely experienced sensory perceptions, synaesthesia, hallucinations, the loss of boundaries and merging with the surrounding world, flashbacks, bad trips, and so on. Again there is a consciousness of these experiences which is usually unreliable, through the so-called distorting mirror (i.e. distorted in time and space) because the physical and ethereal body no longer fit together completely.

However, in general the effects of cannabis will be much "softer" and less strong than those of LSD, though they will become closer to the effects of LSD, as the inhaled THC dose increases: "The effects of high doses of stronger products, hash and hash oil, can be very similar to those of LSD."[42] One example of a very strong hashish experience which was very similar to an LSD experience was that of the American journalist, Bayard Taylor, when he took a very high dose. It started with the experience of part of his ethereal body dissolving in the ethereal world, distorted in time and space. "Suddenly I lost the sense of limitations and restrictions of the senses of flesh and blood. The walls of my body burst outwards and collapsed, and without being able to conceive of the idea of form, I felt that I was taking up a gigantic space. The blood which was pumping through my heart accelerated countless kilometres until it reached my hands and feet. The air which I sucked into my lungs expanded to become seas of clear ether, and the dome of my skull stretched out wider than the firmament of heaven. Bottomless chasms of indescribable blue yawned; clouds passed by which were driven on by the celestial wind and the disc of the sun glowed there. Although I was not thinking about this at all at the time, it was as though the secret of the omnipresence of God was being revealed to me." But then the experience changed to become a bad trip: "I had passed through the paradise of hashish and was then immediately cast down into the most terrible hell ... The blood which had been released stormed through my body like a raging sea. It spurted into my eyes so that I could no longer see; it tolled dully in my ears and banged so hard in my heart that I was afraid that my ribs would break under the blows. I ripped open my shirt, placed my hand on my chest, and tried to count my heartbeats. But there were two hearts, one beating a thousand times per minute, while the other only beat slowly and sluggishly. I thought that my throat was filled with blood up to the top, and that the blood was streaming out of my ears. I could feel the warm blood flowing down my neck and chest. I fled from the room in deep despair, close to madness."[43]

This was an example of an exceptionally strong hashish experience, caused mainly by the partial separation of the ethereal body from the physical body.

The study of the influence of marijuana/hashish on *the will* and on the user's behaviour reveals the following aspects.

As we noted above, in the description of the start of the high induced by marijuana/hashish, the partial separation of the astral body, which rises up, expands, and then becomes slack and relaxed, results in the physical and ethereal body which remains behind becoming indolent, relaxed (with slack muscles) and as heavy as a stone – hence "stoned". The user feels relaxed, and the mari-juana/hashish to some extent works as a tranquillizer. However, particularly during the first part of the high, the situation is rather unstable because the astral forces which have been released can also forcibly become connected with the musculature of the limbs. This gives rise to exactly the opposite condition, and the user becomes rather restless and screwed up. However, this active aspect usually disappears again after a while, especially when the high lasts a long time and the user calms down. Because of the general tendency of the astral body to float up and away from the body, he becomes increasingly calm and passive. Eventually he may even be overcome by apathy, become introspective, and even "absent". Because of the break between the astral body and the physical body, the living force of the will in the soul (astral body) finds it more and more difficult to use the physical body to carry out the will and complete a task. It is as though the physical body is too far removed; it lies "below", heavy, indolent, stoned, and relaxed, without the energy for any conscious action. This phenomenon of increasing passivity can be further accentuated by the increasing dreaminess and sleepiness of consciousness, so that the user finds it more and more difficult to act purposefully and with awareness. We will examine this in greater detail under the heading "Becoming increasingly dreamy and sleepy" (page 108).

To summarize, it is clear that the user increasingly turns in on himself, particularly when he takes a high dose. He withdraws into himself and his own inner world (which includes sensory percep-tions, images and ideas), and this is where he has the experiences produced by the high. His consciousness often becomes dreamier, and unless the extra astral forces which have been released force him to, he will not easily be persuaded to be active. Physically this withdrawal into himself and into his own inner astral world, in which external actions decline, can be seen in the pale colour of the face and the coldness of the body, particularly at the extremities. Van Epen described that "users often feel cold and frequently shiver. The fingers, toes and tip of the nose feel particularly cold."[44] The user's self, carried by the astral body, withdraws from the world of action; it becomes connected to the autonomic nervous system, undergoes the inner process of fusing with other users, and experiences sensory perceptions, images and thoughts in the self with a content of feeling. It is turned inwards; the will to turn, actively and without coercion, to the outside world and to be active in the outside world, becomes weaker and weaker as a result of the partial separation between the astral body on the one hand, and the physical and ethereal body on the other hand.

Changes in the sense of space and time

These were discussed in detail in the description of the effects of LSD. When the physical body (spatial organism), on the one hand, and the ethereal body (the temporal organism), astral body and self, on the other hand, separate, the contents of consciousness can no longer be reflected in the correct dimensions of space and time: the healthy feeling for space and time disappears. William Burroughs wrote: "One more thing about weed (marijuana). Anyone who is under the influence of marijuana is completely unfit to drive a car. Weed distorts your sense of time, and as a result your feeling for spatial relations. Once in New Orleans I had to park my car at the side of the road and sit and wait until the effects of the weed had worn off. I wasn't able to estimate how far away things were, or when I had to turn a corner, or brake at a crossroads."[45]

Becoming increasingly dreamy and sleepy

We characterized the consciousness of the LSD user as a waking dream; this is because of the unpredictability and uncontrolled nature of the experiences which pass in front of the waking consciousness of the tripper like a stream of inner perceptions, images, feelings and ideas. This also applies to someone who uses cannabis. He never knows in advance exactly what will happen to him, or which of the many possible experiences will predominate. In any case, he is at their mercy. Thus it is a waking dream, which is like standing in a stream of inner images etc. and yet it is not like dreaming when you are asleep, but being awake and conscious.

However, this changes, for in the course of a marijuana/hashish-induced high, the user's consciousness can become increasingly dreamy and sleepy, particularly when a high dose has been taken, so that eventually he almost imperceptibly falls into a deep sleep. In this case, he is "out of it", as users say, which means he has moved out of the body, or in even more precise terms, his astral body and Self have separated from the physical and ethereal body, which stays behind asleep on earth.

The in-between stage is the dreamy state of consciousness which was described earlier. Here, because of the *partial* separation of his astral body and Self from the physical and ethereal body, which was brought about by the drug, the user finds himself in a state between waking and sleeping. He is in a sort of dream state which is often considered pleasant and sweet, because of the partially experienced sleeping aspect of consciousness, particularly when a (very) high dose has been taken. This applies to an even greater extent with the use of opium. Rudolf Steiner wrote: "... because he is in his body in such a way (when opium is taken) that he is asleep and at the same time awake. This means that he can enjoy the sweet feeling and this gives him a great sense of wellbeing. It is as though the whole body is permeated with sugar, a special sort of sugar that is thoroughly sweet. However, at the same time, his astral body is free from the physical body, and with this he perceives all sorts of things, though not very clearly. He does not have ordinary dreams, but sees the spiritual world. He makes long journeys through the spiritual world... The people of the East have many things which they communicate from the spiritual world, albeit incorrectly, thanks to the use of opium, *hashish* etc."[46] The communications are incorrect, partly as a result of a partial separation between the physical and ethereal body, so that astral perceptions are often distorted in the distorting mirror of consciousness. (See the effects of LSD, p. 52 et seq.)

To summarize, it may be said that the astral body of the user is forced by the effect of cannabis to be gradually separated from the physical and ethereal body, and is then assimilated into the cosmic astral world, where it has all sorts of spiritual experiences in a dreamy state of consciousness, though these are distorted and unreliable. Eventually the user loses consciousness and really falls asleep; his astral body has then withdrawn completely from the physical and ethereal body and, until the user wakes up, remains in the cosmic, astral world (in addition to the connection which it has with the system of the spinal cord).

This brings us to the final stage of the marijuana/hashish high, which may take place, viz., falling asleep and sleep itself.

Falling asleep

Obviously we can be brief about this. The user may almost imperceptibly fall asleep, following an immobile state when his eyes are closed and he is turned inwards, particularly when he has taken a high dose. This means that his astral body connects in the abovementioned way with the nerves of the system of the spinal cord and dissolves like an astral drop in the cosmic astral sea; his ethereal body and physical body are left behind on earth, relaxed and asleep. However, this last stage by no means always occurs; many users do not let it come to this.

The hangover

After the high, many users, particularly chronic users, may find that they are troubled by a "hangover" to a greater or lesser extent i.e. in extreme cases, "a constant sense of indifference, lack of interest and listless apathy which may last for days, and sometimes for more than a week, accompanied by a very pleasant (relaxed) physical condition."[47] *Handbuch der Rauschdrogen* (The Handbook of Hallucinogenic Drugs) describes how "the user becomes aware of the loss of spiritual energy in the form of exhaustion, tiredness and not being able to get moving."[48] This is easy to imagine, because the intense dreaming consciousness induced by the drug overwhelms the user with such an unusually vehement abundance of experiences that his inner Self must operate on a much higher number of revolutions than normal. He therefore becomes inwardly exhausted, empty and depleted. In addition, his astral body will have some difficulty returning completely to the physical body, particularly in the case of regular use. This could be because metabolic traces of cannabis remain in the human body for so long. In short, the user cannot go back into his body immediately, but remains hanging slightly above it, not quite there. This explains his dreaminess and slightly absent-minded mood. It also explains the tepid, indifferent and uninterested mood which often prevails with regard to earthly and practical matters, following repeated use. It is self-evident that these moods can lead to enormous problems, particularly at school which requires attention and effort!

This brings us to the end of our description of the course of a marijuana/hashish high. The user often starts with a great high, and may finish by falling asleep. Afterwards he may find that he has a hangover, particularly in the case of regular use, and then uses the drug as a possible way of escaping the tepid, empty, listless mood. This brings us to the question of the consequences of regular use, and after a while, of chronic use.

The consequences of chronic marijuana/hashish use

One of the first consequences for the health of a chronic cannabis user lies in the fact that his astral body partially withdraws from the ethereal or physical body during the many highs which last between two and four hours. This means that the forces of the astral body and of the Self during the hours of use are much less able to have a formative effect on the more or less undifferentiated growth of the ethereal body. "Normal growth" is the result of two processes: the reproduction of cells brought about by the ethereal forces and, structural formation brought about by the forces of the astral body and the Self, so that the ethereal forces are converted into *creative forces*." (Victor Bott, *Anthroposophical Medicine*).[49] It is these creative forces which are lacking as a result of the partial separation of the astral body and the Self from the ethereal body. The growth and structure of the physical body are therefore in danger of acquiring a less human/individual character; during the high, undifferentiated growth processes can take over and flourish. An abnormal and unhealthy formation of substance may develop, interfering with the healthy structure of the physical body.

This can be seen most clearly in the creation/structure and formation of reproductive material and heredity, as this is easily and quickly affected. Some facts are given below by way of illustration:

- In men: potency declines with chronic use of cannabis. The number of sperm in the semen is lower than normal, and the mobility of the sperm is reduced;[50] in contrast, the number of abnormal sperm actually clearly increases.[51]
- In women: girls who smoke marijuana three times a week for a period of six months are more likely to have abnormal menstrual cycles, without ovulation, in comparison with girls of the same age who do not use the drug. In addition, there is a reduction in the prolactin content, which could have an effect on the production of mother's milk.[50] According to research at the Institute of Sexual Behaviour by Masters and Johnson in St. Louis, the female "hormone regulation" is seriously affected by the influence of marijuana.[51]
- In pregnant women: THC passes through the placenta and affects the development of the unborn child. In a recent large-scale study published in the *New England Journal of Medicine* (23 March 1989), a research team from Boston came to the following conclusion: "The use of marijuana proved to cause a reduction in birth weight of 79 grammes, and a reduction in body length of 0.5 cm. (with the use of cocaine, these reductions were 93 grammes and 0.7 cm.)."[52]

Tests on animals show that a high THC content in the mother leads to abnormalities in the embryo.[53] THC has been found in human mother's milk.[50]

– In men and women: damage to the chromosomes is likely. Animal tests showed that marijuana/hashish slows down the process of cell division and inhibits the formation of DNA, the building block of the chromosomes.[51] Three doses of hashish corresponding to the contents of three joints per week for a period of three years irreparably damage the chromosomes of animals.[53]

Thus we see that the chronic use of cannabis has serious consequences for the harmonious and healthy structure of the user's physical body. It can also influence the effectiveness of the immune system. In this respect, Van Epen wrote: "Animal tests showed that when a large dose of cannabis is given, this results in a decline in the operation of the immune system. This effect has not been clearly shown in human beings. Recently this field of research has been of particular interest because the notorious new disease, AIDS, involves a reduction or even complete absence of the immune system. It seems likely that the use of marijuana would have an adverse effect on AIDS patients and those who are HIV positive."[54]

The above was a description of the effects of the chronic use of cannabis on the user's physical health. We will continue by looking at the influence which it has on his psychological state.

In this context, an examination of the human *soul* containing the forces of thinking, feeling and the will, reveals the following effects: because the periods that the user is high start taking up a significant part of his life, the changes in his thinking, feeling and will which occur during these periods will increasingly influence the quality of these spiritual forces themselves.

The following pattern emerges:

– *Thinking* becomes increasingly confused, associative and dreamy, even at times when the drug is not used. The logical thread disappears, there is a loss of memory and a decline in concentration, typical of a hash smoker. In addition, metabolic traces of THC build up in the fatty tissue of the brain (in the case of chronic use) and form a sort of store which increases in size every time the drug is used. (55) This means that the brain is no longer able to fulfil its task as an instrument for creating consciousness for active thinking directed by the Self.

— *Feeling*: following a surfeit of feelings experienced while he is high, the chronic user often feels rather hollow, empty and bleak emotionally as soon as the effect of the drug wears off. You often hear chronic users say things like: "All my feelings are grey. I can no longer get in touch with my true feelings." This is actually a reason for them to take marijuana/hashish again, because many users know that it makes them feel something, and it means that something is happening.

— *The will*: the user increasingly lacks any will and the chronic user typically says things like: "I do everything by halves ..."

In addition, an unstable relationship develops between both the astral body in relation to the physical and ethereal body, and the ethereal body in relation to the physical body, as a result of the repeated separations of both the astral body and the ethereal body and the presence of THC traces in the human body.

This means that, when the high comes to an end, the feeling of physical relaxation can make way for the opposite feelings of nervousness, restlessness and fear, which are an expression of the fact that the user's astral body and Self can no longer connect adequately with the physical body, which in turn also has an unstable connection with the ethereal body. The human organism has lost its stability, so that the relationships are incomplete and unstable, leading to inner insecurity and fear. Furthermore, in special circumstances, breaks may take place between these parts of the body which can lead to unexpected highs in cases of stress, tiredness etc. even when the drug is not used, i.e. occurring spontaneously. This flashback was mentioned for LSD, though it is much "softer" in the case of cannabis.

Nevertheless, these effects often constitute a gradual process of which the user is usually unaware, particularly as it may take some people a long time to notice the consequences of the drug – for example, if they have a strong constitution (relationship between the different aspects of the being as a whole), a great deal of vitality, and so on.

In any case, every time that marijuana/hashish is taken, the constituent parts of the being as a whole become more dissolved. The astral body in particular partly dissolves in the astral world and the ethereal body partly dissolves in the ethereal world, while the Self looks on as the constituent parts lose their inner cohesion and strength as a result. Marijuana/hashish has an evaporating effect, partly pulling the person up out of his being, away from the earth and into the cosmos.

What happens when young people regularly smoke cannabis? As we described above, this means that they are going against their own development because these processes of separation, partial death and dreaminess go in the opposite direction from the path which leads towards the earth, towards life, and this is the path which every young person must follow on the road to adulthood.

Although the reasons why many young people use cannabis regularly are very understandable, and although they may consider it as a remedy for their inner problems, it will not help them in the long run. In fact, the use of this drug is more of a replacement for fellow human beings who could also provide feelings of warmth, security, attention, concern, consolation, as well as fascinating experiences. In this light, the desire for the drug is actually a desire for people and for a meaningful encounter with others: at home, at school and in the world. It is a desire for community, a connection with the community of man on earth in the here and now, a desire for community in which others see you and in which you are wanted.

6

Opiates

Before describing the history and effects of opiates, we will begin by recounting the Indian fairy tale about the way in which the poppy, which produces the opiates – opium, morphine, heroin – came into the world.

The fairy tale about the poppy

There was once a holy man who had withdrawn from the world and had built a little hut in the jungle. He meditated there for twenty years and did not speak, until one day he was able to understand the language of animals. His only food was brought to him by a friendly rat, and he did not ask why the rat did this. Every day it would sigh very meaningfully. One day, speaking his first words for twenty years, the holy man asked: "Why do you lament so?" The rat sighed: "Oh, holy man, my life consists of only fear and then even more fear. I am constantly afraid of my greatest enemy, the cat. You cannot understand what a terrible life this is. You are a holy man, and you have become so powerful an ascetic that you could change me into a better creature with a single word, but with all your holiness you don't give a thought to my sad lot." The rat pestered the wise man in this way, until one day he finally did change the rat into a cat – but the rat/cat was no happier. "If only you hadn't changed me into a cat," it constantly complained. "Now I'm always afraid of dogs. But you have ended my life as a rat and have given me this terrible life as a cat. Why don't you change me into a dog? After all, you started all this. Why don't you take the next step?" The cat wouldn't stop bothering him.

However, once the rat-cat was a dog, he was afraid of jackals, and because the master had gone this far, he had to take the next step. Of course, the rat-cat-dog-jackal was afraid of the tiger, so one day the rat became a tiger. He roared and growled ferociously, and all the animals in the jungle cowered whenever they heard him. But one day, the tiger timidly went back to the holy man's hut. "Now what's

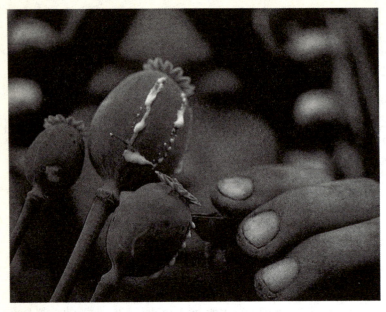

Photograph: Cutting the poppy head to release the juice.

the matter?" asked the holy man. Surely you're not telling me that you're still afraid?" "Of course not," said the rat-tiger, "and yet my heart is burdened with sorrow. I simply got it wrong. A tiger is not the highest creature. I tell you, yesterday I saw the King's elephant. My whiskers stood on end. He was decked with splendid cloths and looked out of this world, and he was carrying a gilt throne where the king was seated in all his glory. I tell you that truly I could never be happy as a tiger, now that I've seen this. You must change me into an elephant."

The holy man was furious, but the rat was right – because he had started fulfilling the rat's wishes, he now had to change him into an elephant. The great creature first trampled on his hut, and then walked away through the jungle. After some time he returned, and apologised profusely, saying: "Oh dear, again I got everything wrong. I was captured and taken to the King's court, where I was tamed. It was terrible, but I allowed them to do anything they wanted, and I was given magnificent trappings. But the King did not want to mount me, and had the Queen sit on my throne. Then I was overcome with despair, because I understood that the highest creature there is, is a queen. So I threw off my throne, trampled on the palace gates, and now I am here. Will you change me into a beautiful girl?" Obviously the holy man did not want to do this, but in the end he did.

When the King went hunting in the jungle, he saw a beautiful girl sitting at the foot of a tree. Obviously he was curious, and asked who the beautiful girl was. The girl wept and moaned: "Oh King, I am a king's daughter who was kidnapped as a little girl. This is how I came to be with the hermit here in the wood. But he did nothing for me. He kept me as a slave, and didn't allow me to leave the wood once. Oh, it's a miserable life."

The rat had always retained his rat character, which means that everything he did was in his own interests, without thinking about others. But the King fell in love with the girl and took her out of the woods on his elephant. She became his favourite wife. Now she had everything she could have dreamed of, and much more. But one night, a moonbeam shone on her bed and told the King's favourite wife that she had come to the end of her life as a rat. Full of fear, she walked around like a rat in a trap and came into the garden. She tried to hide from the moonbeam and dig a hole. She broke her beautiful nails, but it did not do any good.

This is how they found her the next morning, with earth on her scratched and torn hands, and her beautiful face which was now cold. The King was inconsolable, and in his despair he asked the holy man for advice. The latter told him the whole story, and said: "Throw her body into a well, and then fill it with earth. A flower will grow there which will contain consolation, poison and a blessing, all at the same time."

This is how the poppy came into the world.[1]

This wonderful fairy tale reveals a number of themes which very cleverly reflect the essence of what is involved in using opiates. Some of these themes are described below:

– The rat starts on the path of changing his identity because he is afraid: "Oh holy man, my life consists of only fear and then even more fear." This is what he wants to end. Compare these words with: "Heroin has one quality which is the main reason and virtually the only reason that it is taken nowadays by young people. It drives out all fear."[2]

– The rat-cat-dog and so on, which constantly complains, moans and reproaches, and plays on the holy man's feelings, putting pressure on him, behaves in a way that is very similar to the yearning opium addict (or to any drug addict in general), who will do anything so that he can get his dope on time. Van Epen wrote: "A junkie (opium addict) is prepared to do virtually anything to get his fix. He will lie and steal, blackmail and manipulate, and try anything to persuade the doctor to write him a prescription. In doing so, he will be very cunning, not going to his own doctor but to one who is on call for the weekend, and will say that his own doctor always gives him this prescription which he needs. If the doctor refuses, he may threaten suicide, or less often, become aggressive. It will be impossible to get him out of the waiting room until he gets his way. Once the doctor has relented, he will become an easier victim the following weekend. Once the doctor has written a few prescriptions, the junkie will undoubtedly blame him for causing his addiction. This will then be used as an argument for extorting even more prescriptions."[3]

The fairy tale reflects these characteristics of an addiction to opiates in a very striking way, and shows how a person who is originally merely anxious can be transformed into a dissatisfied, insatiable, selfish user who manipulates others.

– The holy man succumbed. "Of course the holy man didn't want to do it, but he did it anyway." Just as so many parents, family members, friends and acquaintances of the addict also succumb. The latter will not thank them for this. On the contrary, he is only using them. In many cases he will even steal first from the very people who helped him and cared about him most. "The great creature first trampled on the holy man's hut, and then walked away through the jungle."

Each time the rat's new identity only satisfied him for a little while, only made him happy for a moment. This also applies to the euphoria produced by opiates. For a relatively short while there is no fear, restlessness or sorrow, but warmth, a sense of satisfaction and peace. Then it is gone again, and the fear and pain (of the withdrawal symptoms), and the desire for more, return.

These were some of the images from the fairy tale. Obviously this description is by no means complete, but the examples show how much wisdom the fairy tale contains. It ends: "This is how the poppy came into the world."

We will now look at the background of the opiates from the perspective of history. We will begin with a description of the history of opium, and then devote some attention to the history of morphine, a product derived from opium, and subsequently of heroin, which is prepared from morphine.

History of the opiates

Opium

The first mention of the plant from which opium is derived, *Papava somniferum* (see photograph on p.116) can be found on a Sumerian clay tablet dating from approximately 3500 BC, on which the poppy is described in cuneiform script as a sleep-inducing and narcotic drug. The plant is indicated with the signs, Gil and Hull. The Sumerians also called it the plant of joy.

From Sumeria, the knowledge of opium spread to Ancient Egypt, where it was used, amongst other things, as a "remedy to pacify children who cried excessively" (approximately 1600 BC). However, opium was known not only for its narcotic properties, but also as a drug which produced dangerous dreams and induced sleep. On the tombstone of an Egyptian physician, in approximately 800 BC, the plant was praised with the following words: "Plant at the gates of night and death, taking away sorrow and knowledge, granting dreams, sleep and death."[4]

It is not entirely inconceivable that opium also played a role as an ingredient in the so-called "drink of oblivion" which was an important substance during the initiation ritual into the Mysteries, as we shall see later in this chapter (see footnote 55). However, we cannot be certain of this.

In Ancient Greece the poppy was specially dedicated to three gods: to Thanatos, the god of death, to his brother, Hypnos, the god of sleep, and to the latter's son, Morpheus, the god of dreams (hence the word "morphine"). Representations of these three gods were often bedecked with garlands of poppies.

In the *Odyssey*, it was probably opium from Egypt which was celebrated as the magic potion mixed into the wine to "erase anxiety, heartache and the memory of any suffering. Anyone who took this no longer had tears on his face all day, even if his father and mother had died, even if his own brother or dearest son were killed before his very eyes."[5] It is striking that for this reason, opium has also been called "the hibernation of feelings". In medicine it has often been used as an anaesthetic and painkiller.

During the Roman Empire, opium was often used as a painkiller, as a sleeping remedy, and to a lesser extent, merely as a stimulant. In this respect, in the 1st century AD, Petronius wrote : "And he took many sweet pills made of poppy juice which promised joy and peaceful rest." However, people also often committed suicide with the help of opium.

Opium was also known during the Byzantine and Islamic Empires. In approximately 750 AD, Theoditus of Smyrna wrote: "Only the dregs of society and those without possessions or rights surrender to opium. They use it as a remedy against their inferiority. However, for honourable and respected citizens, it is used as a medicine in the case of illness."[7]

Persia was the country where poppies were cultivated on the largest scale in the Islamic world. From there, opium spread to the east and its medicinal uses even reached China via India. However, it was not used on any significant scale there because, in China, acupuncture was used as an efficient method of controlling pain. This was quite different in the Islamic world where the use of alcohol was forbidden by the prophet Mohammed but the use of opium and hashish was not. In fact, from the early Middle Ages, Arab doctors prescribed opium on a large scale for medical purposes. One of the greatest Arab scholars of the time, Avicenna, who himself died of opium poisoning in 1037, introduced the remedy to European physicians. From the 12th century it was increasingly used in

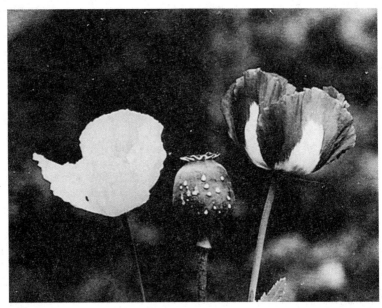

Photograph: Flowering poppies and an unripe cut ovary with milky juice.

European medicine. Paracelsus, the famous Renaissance physician, who lived from 1493 to 1541, used opium as an ingredient in his well-known "miracle cure", laudanum, a painkiller and tranquillizer which was used in many households until our own century.

In *Europe*, the use of opium as a popular stimulant dates from the end of the 18th century. Its popularity quickly spread amongst all classes of society in England in the 19th century and, above all, amongst the poor industrial workers and dockers. With reference to this, Thomas de Quincey wrote: "Three notable apothecaries in London ... told me ... that there are an enormous number of opium eaters. When I came to Manchester a few years later, several cotton mill owners told me that the custom of eating opium was becoming prevalent amongst the workers; Saturday – at the end of the after-noon – packets of one or two grains of opium (approximately 65 mg.) were piling up on the counters of the apothecaries. These had been prepared in advance for taking in the evening. The reason given for this was the miserable wages which did not allow the workers to buy beer or gin."[8]

In France, opium also became popular, though to a lesser extent, especially in the ports. However, it was not eaten or drunk as in England, but was smoked. This habit had been taken over from the Chinese.

This brings us to an important and tragic phase in the history of the use of opium, viz., the large-scale use which developed in China in the course of the 19th century.

In *China*, opium had been smoked on a small scale from the beginning of the 17th century. The custom was probably taken over from the Arabs. As its use gradually increased over the years, it became economically profitable for England, the largest trading nation at the time, to meet the increasing demand. For this purpose, extensive poppy fields were planted in India (Bengal). The English East India Company was awarded a trading monopoly and it started to export more opium to China than was required to meet the demand. In other words, they started to "push" it, to use the modern expression. This had the following result: the trade rose from several thousand chests of opium in 1773 to approximately 30,000 chests in 1837. China was opposed to this, and prohibited the importation of opium in 1794, but this did not do any good. The English got round the prohibitions and an extremely lucrative trade in smuggling opium flourished in the ports of the Chinese Empire. In 1839, the

Chinese government, which had been shocked by the disastrous consequences of the use of opium, with the emaciated addicts who wasted away and eventually died, sent a government commissioner to Canton to put an end to these clandestine practices. This government commissioner, who was called Lin, didn't waste any time. He seized more than 20,000 English chests of opium (over 1000 tons) and had them destroyed. Then he introduced the death penalty for trading in opium. In addition, he threatened to seize English ships if the prohibition were violated. England literally responded as follows: "With this demand the Chinese government has definitively destroyed every sense of safety (the safety to engage in free trade)."[9] Following a short period of skirmishes, this resulted in "war". It raged from 1840-1842. The military powers of the Chinese Empire, with its population of 370 million at the time, primitively armed with flintlock rifles and so on, confronted the army of 10,000 soldiers sent by the English government, who were armed with extremely modern weapons including machine guns. It was an unequal fight. The Chinese were unable to stand up to them and capitulated in 1842. England demanded compensation for the 20,000 chests of opium destroyed by Lin, was given free access to five important Chinese ports, and Hong Kong became a British colony.

The Second Opium War raged from 1856-60. England, France and America forced China to reduce the state of isolation even further and to increase trade with the west. More Chinese ports were opened for the trade in opium, amongst other things. The Chinese authorities were forced to abandon their moral stance against opium consumption, and realized "that the current generation of opium smokers want opium and must have it."[10] The drug was legalized and great profits were made from it: 8% tax on the value. There was a dramatic increase in the number of addicts: from 2 million in 1850 to 20 million in 1878. Millions of people died as a result of their opium addiction. In 1880, the opium imported from India reached a peak of 6,500 tons. This was a reason for China itself to start growing poppies on a large scale. The Chinese produced their own opium, which competed for quality with the Indian variety. It was very successful, and by the turn of the century imports from India had fallen to 2,300 tons, while domestic production had risen to 22,000 tons.

Emaciated people who were wasting away were now seen daily in the large cities, but by far the majority of addicts did not let it come to this. In order to prevent any loss of face, people would commit suicide by taking an overdose before reaching the last stages of addiction.

The capitulation treaty of 1860 contained a clause which stated that foreign missionaries could settle in China. On the one hand, the situation they found in China in terms of the loss of human dignity resulting from the forced principle of free trade stimulated them to try and find a way to help the opium addicts. On the other hand, it filled them with a deep moral revulsion for the politics of free trade, obviously insofar as this related to the free trade in opium. A rich Quaker missionary who founded the company for the suppression of the opium trade in 1874, introduced the motto: "What is morally bad cannot be politically good."[11] This company subsequently lobbied extensively in England to achieve its goal. It pressurized the British government to send a Royal Commission to study opium. In 1896, this produced a report stating that a prohibition on opium would be an intolerable burden on the Indian government and would not help China either. Furthermore, the Asiatics, in contrast with whites, "were largely immune to the negative consequences of opium".[12] There was great disappointment in the anti-opium lobby. However, it persevered, and gained increasing support in America when Chinese immigrant labourers, who had been brought to the west of the United States to work on the construction of the transcontinental railway, surrendered to opium on a massive scale, particularly once they became unemployed. The Americans shuddered to see the consequences of opium addiction, and issued strict laws prohibiting the smoking of opium. This was fairly easy, because a large part of the population already had a strong moral stance against the use of alcohol. In fact, the use of alcohol had been prohibited in a number of states from the middle of the 19th century, ever since the Puritans had started campaigning against it in the early 1800s.

However, there were also purely political and economic reasons for opposing the use of opium on a massive scale. The United States had "liberated" the Philippines from the Spanish just before the turn of the century, where they had discovered how extensive the scourge could be: approximately 40% of the adult population had become addicted,[13] and the competing colonial powers (England and France) made a lot of money from it. In 1906, Theodore Roosevelt, president of the United States, wrote: "By acting against the opium trade we are improving our position in Asia in two respects. Those who suffer under it become our natural allies, and moreover, we are weakening the economy of the colonial powers."[13] Under the banner: "It is the sacred duty of the United States to bring the peoples of the world freedom and the possibility of a good life",[14] he formulated three key points of his foreign policy: a) opium is a serious problem in Asia; b) the United States must support China at the broadest international level (in fact, the widowed Chinese empress had issued strict laws against the use of opium in that year, though without any significant effect), and c) the United States should champion the general prohibition of opium throughout the world.

In the same year (1906), under pressure from the British and the international anti-opium lobby, as well as the political developments outlined above, the British parliament unanimously accepted a motion charging the government "to take the necessary steps to bring a rapid end to the opium trade between India and China."[15]

In the following ten years, at the instigation of the United States and China, there were three international conferences aimed at the fight against smuggling, the strict regulation of the trade in opium and opiates and the restriction of production for medicinal purposes. The English and Chinese governments started co-operating to control consumption in China. England reduced the importation of opium from India at the same rate that China destroyed its poppy plantations. In 1917, China destroyed the last chests of Indian opium. This brought an end to the official English opium trade for non-medical purposes.

The International Opium Treaty of The Hague (1912) and subsequent conferences provided that henceforth all non-clandestine opium and opiates should be under strict international control. Production could take place only for medical purposes. However, it was to be some time before the legislation was in any sense watertight and most countries had actually signed the treaty. The process came to a temporary end with the 1925 Geneva Opium Treaty. (The next treaties were not concluded until 1961 and 1971.) However, the state of affairs was extremely unsatisfactory: the American and Chinese delegations left the conference early, completely disillusioned because they did not consider the regulations sufficiently radical, and thought that without any stringent prohibitions it was impossible to counteract the opium plague. (By way of illustration: in 1925, the gross income for the Netherlands for the opium trade was no less than 36,621,000 florins; in 1938, this income was still 11,948,000 florins. These were sums which the colonial treasury could hardly do without at the time, so that people were not very fussy about imposing strict rules.)[16]

Thus the problems continued to exist, particularly for China. The central government increasingly lost control of the disintegrating empire. In political terms, the regional leaders started to hold power and discovered that there was a great deal of money to be earned from the production and trade of opium. The use of opium survived in China on a large scale until the early 1950s. It was only when the Communists, led by Mao Tse Tung, decided to impose strict controls and actually implemented this decision very thoroughly, that both the illegal trade and the use of the drug in China were completely eradicated. As a result there was virtually no opium problem in China until fairly recently. However, in the last few years more and more reports indicate that the use of opium, and now also of heroin, is being revived. According to an estimate in an internal Chinese police report, there were 300,000 opium and heroin addicts in 1991; the official figure given is 70,000.[17]

In the rest of the world the use of opium has also drastically decreased but morphine and, later, heroin, have proved themselves to be "worthy" replacements, as we shall see.

To conclude this historical account of opium, we should explain what is really is. What is the substance known as opium and how is it prepared?

Opium is made from the sap of *Papaver somniferum* (opium poppy), a plant in the poppy family which also includes our own common poppy. The traditional method of extracting opium is described below. When the flower has blossomed, the unripe seed cases are superficially scored with a knife, so that the white juice flows out of the cut. When it is exposed to the air, it dries up in the form of a malleable substance which turns brown. This substance is scratched off the seed cases with a blunt knife. This is the so-called "raw" opium. It still contains all sorts of impurities which can be removed by certain purification methods. This produces so-called "smoking" opium. In his *Opium, Diary of a Cure*, Jean Cocteau described the following purification method: "I recommend adding a litre of old wine to the water in which the raw ball is soaking. Avoid boiling it, and filter it seven times in the space of eight days."[18]

Raw opium has a bitter taste and an intoxicating odour. It contains 25 active ingredients (alkaloids), in which the toxic morphine accounts for by far the greatest part of the total composition (10–14%). The most important other active ingredients, which jointly account

for between 5.5 and 10.8% of the total composition, are:
- codeine (a cough remedy which works more or less like morphine);
- papaverine, (a toxic substance which relaxes and relieves cramps; it affects the smooth musculature of the intestines, oesophagus and gall bladder);
- narcotine, (a toxic substance which relaxes; it works more or less like papaverine);
- narceine, (a powerful painkiller which has a strong effect on the smooth musculature);
- thebaine, (a toxin which causes cramps).

The above shows that the various constituent parts of opium on the one hand reinforce each other and, on the other hand, at least partially, counteract each other. This explains why the effect of raw opium, which is actually based primarily on the effect of the morphine it contains, is still rather different from, the effect of pure, refined morphine. When raw opium is purified for smoking, the percentage of morphine in relation to the other alkaloids increases, so that the effect of smoking opium is stronger than that of raw opium. However, it does not achieve the strength of effect of pure morphine.

Morphine

Even before the end of the eighteenth century, research had been carried out in virtually every country in Europe to discover the active ingredient in the substance known as opium. The question was whether one or more substances could be found in opium which were responsible for its effects. In the early years of chemistry a great deal of work was done on this question and, by the turn of the century, there was a feeling in scientific circles that a discovery was imminent.

However, surprisingly, it was the twenty-year-old pharmacist's apprentice, F.W. Serturner, who was the first to isolate the most active component in opium in 1803 in Paderborn, Germany. He dissolved the raw opium in distilled water, heated it and then processed it, inter alia, with ammoniac, which produced a sediment consisting of a new, white, crystalline substance. He wondered whether this substance might be responsible for the consciousness-changing properties of opium. In order to investigate this, he sprinkled the white powder on a hunk of bread and gave it to a stray dog to eat. Serturner noted: "After eating the substance, the dog soon fell asleep and then vomited. When it had some more, everything was vomited up, but the tendency to sleep persisted for several hours. Therefore this substance is the true narcotic ingredient in opium."[19] Subsequently he tried again with a neighbour's dog. This time he was not so lucky: "The creature lolled about in a drunken sleep and finally died."[19] He also did controlled tests. After removing the crystalline substance which he had isolated, he fed the remaining substance to a small dog, and had a mouse breathe in the gases released during the preparation. Neither of these creatures responded in any way, and therefore Serturner believed that he could conclude with certainty that the great stimulating effect of opium was based not on resinous or extracted elements, but was caused by this special crystallized substance.[19] He called this "morphine" after the Greek god Morpheus.

Two years later in 1805, after carrying out several experiments on himself and some other young people, he published his discovery in the form of a letter to the *Journal der Pharmacie* in Leipzig, but he was not taken very seriously. In 1806, 1811 and 1817 he wrote more articles. In the last of these he described the alkaline salt-forming properties of morphine. It was because of this that vegetable substances with these properties were later called alkaloids.

For a long time Serturner complained that the importance of his discovery had not been recognized. However, in 1817, he was accepted as an extraordinary member of the Society for General Mineralogy in Jena. This was a great honour, particularly as the record was signed by the chairman of the society, Goethe. The latter was also responsible – presumably pulling strings behind the scenes – for the fact that in the same year the pharmacist Serturner was granted an honourary doctorate at the University of Jena.

Serturner's discovery had far-reaching consequences: on the one hand, it had the result that in the course of time the other alkaloids contained in raw opium were traced (codeine, papaverine, narcotine etc.). On the other hand, it was hoped that morphine would be a substance which would not be addictive, while it would still have a similar effect to opium if the right dose were taken. To study this, it was prescribed to opium addicts as a substitute. Their hopes were fulfilled and the addicts stopped taking opium, but after a while they could no longer do without morphine. Therefore the problem had merely moved elsewhere.

At that time it was believed that the feeling of "opium hunger" was caused by the organ where the feeling of hunger was situated, i.e. by the stomach, and it was argued that if the substance could be introduced into the body "past the stomach", the hunger for opium or morphine would no longer exist. How could this be achieved? The solution came with the invention of syringes for giving injections.

In 1864 the pharmacist Charles-Gabriël Pravaz came up with this solution when he saw a rat catcher who was spraying awkward nooks and crannies with poison with his large hand syringe. That was it. Two days later he had assembled a much smaller version of the syringe with a long hollow needle at the front. A week later, six opium addicts presented themselves for an experiment with injections of morphine: after this, none of them ever again took laudanum, which contained opium. It was thought that this might be the solution: a subcutaneous injection of morphine with the anaesthetizing and painkilling properties of opium with the result that there could be no more "opium hunger" or addiction.

However, a few years later during the Franco-Prussian War of 1870-1871, these hopes were disappointed. Morphine had been injected on a large scale to relieve the pain of the wounded, and during operations and amputations. It became clear that when they had been repeatedly given morphine, many wounded soldiers felt a growing desire for the drug, even though it was no longer necessary from the point of view of relieving pain. After the war many soldiers started to inject morphine themselves, using it merely as a stimulant and to produce feelings of warmth, relaxation, oblivion and happiness.

This was morphine addiction on a large scale, and the first empirical studies of this condition were published in the 1890s. It was found that there were many addicts amongst doctors and pharmacists. Half of the 47 addicts discovered in these professions, in a study carried out at that time, had become addicted to morphine "to tolerate the burdens of the profession, which was so involved with human suffering."[20]

Following experiences in the United States, where morphine had become a popular drug after the end of the American Civil War (1861-1865), the drug was prohibited by the international Opium Treaties of 1912 (and later) because of its addictive properties. This did not apply when it was used for medical purposes. However, this did not mean that the use of morphine as a drug disappeared. Because of its euphoric properties, its use and the addiction to it have continued to the present day, particularly among doctors, the nursing profession and pharmacists (who have easy access to it).

Heroin

The intensive search continued for an ideal substance, i.e. a pain-killer which both relieved pain and was non-addictive. In 1898, it was again thought that this had been found. In the Bayer pharmaceutical factory (Germany), the thirty-seven-year-old Professor Heinrich Dreser produced a substance (diacetyl*morphine*) based on morphine, by adding acetic acid and carrying out complicated purification procedures, including a procedure with ether. After a short period of experimentation – barely two months – he concluded that this substance had the following properties:[21]

- In contrast with the sleep-inducing properties of morphine, it acts more as a stimulant.
- It dispels any feeling of fear.
- The very smallest dose suppresses the coughing reflex, even in patients with TB.
- Morphine addicts treated with this substance immediately lose all interest in morphine.

After his death, Dreser was described by the Bayer company as "a true scholar, with a rather sharp, original personality. He was not easy to get on with, nor very sociable. He remained aloof from his colleagues and it was difficult to persuade him to attend meetings or conferences."[21] This was the man who thought that he had discovered the ultimate miracle drug. All it needed was a catchy name. This became "heroin", after the Greek *heros* (hero), because of the heroic qualities ascribed to the new drug.

In the annual letters sent to doctors (the "Bayer Bible") the company introduced heroin as follows: "A substance with properties which are non-addictive, which is easy to use, and which is the only substance which can provide a lightning cure for morphine addicts."[21] In the same year (1898) Bayer started a large-scale, worldwide campaign in all the major newspapers for its two new miracle drugs: aspirin and heroin (the perfect remedy for coughs).

Heroin was now sold on a large scale all over the world. However, in 1904 the Frenchman, Morel-Lavallée, challenging Bayer's good reputation, dared to state that heroin certainly was addictive. A year later he discovered that, in the blood, heroin quickly changes to morphine, so that the effect of morphine is doubled. Dreser had considered this hypothetically impossible, as the chemical formulae of morphine and heroin are very different. In 1912, Bayer decided to stop the weekly advertisements and, in the same year, because of the increasing heroin addiction, particularly in the United States, heroin was placed on the list of prohibited substances (for non-medical use) of the International Opium Treaty of The Hague.

Although heroin was recognized as an addictive drug, it was still prescribed, particularly in the United States, as medication for opium addiction, because it was considered to be a much less harmful drug than opium. It was only in 1924, when heroin addiction began to assume epidemic proportions in the United States, that it was also prohibited there in the form of medication. In many other countries the use of heroin continued on quite a large scale for a long time. In 1925 in Egypt, for example, many businessmen paid their workers part of their weekly wages in the form of heroin pills.

Heroin went "underground" as a result of the international prohibitions. After a time, criminal organizations took over the production, trade and sales and, since the beginning of the current wave of heroin addiction in the late 1960s and early 1970s, they have been earning gigantic sums of money from it. Heroin was, and still is, refined in a very pure form from raw opium in clandestine laboratories in the so-called "Golden Triangle" (the border area of Burma, Thailand, Laos and China), and also in Pakistan, Afghanistan and Turkey. From these countries the drug is taken to its destination via special smuggling routes, and it is then cut (e.g. with lactose) by dealers and middlemen. As a result, the heroin, which was originally virtually pure, is generally only 20-60% pure in the end.[22] En route the price has mushroomed: the price at which the heroin is sold (the so-called "street value") is often thousands of times what it cost to produce.

Since the present wave of heroin addiction there has been an enormous increase in the number of addicts: the drug is used as a remedy to drive out fear, sorrow, (inner) pain, rage and depression, and for many, usually young, people, it has become an essential drug if life is to be at all bearable.

The effects of opiates

The effects of opium

As a starting point for the description of the effects of opium, we will quote a well-known description of an opium trance given by S. Hedayat:

"I wanted to concentrate, and only the delicate smoke of opium could bring my thoughts together and grant me peace.

I smoked the opium I had left, so that this miracle-producing drug would remove all the obstacles and veils from my eyes and drive out all the towering, distant and ashen memories piled up in front of me. The state I had waited for came to me even more strongly than I had hoped: slowly my thoughts assumed great clarity and a delicate purity. I fell into a state which was half-sleep and half-impotence.

Then it was as though a great weight had been removed from my chest. It seemed to me that the law of gravity no longer applied to me, and I could fly freely after my thoughts, which were rich, wide-ranging and absolutely clear. I was filled with a deep sense of indescribable well-being. I was freed from the burden of my body. My whole being felt as though it had been assimilated into the silently growing world of plants in a tranquil form of existence which was yet full of enchantingly lovely forms and colours.

The interrelationship between my thoughts disappeared and they combined with their forms and colours. I was submerged in waves of the softest tenderness. I could feel the beating of my heart and my pulse. All of this was full of the deepest significance, and at the same time filled me with an infinite sense of wonder. I wanted to surrender completely to this sleep of oblivion.

Oh, if only this total oblivion were possible, if only it could be permanent. My eyes, closing, transcending sleep, dived down into the absolute void and I was no longer aware of my existence; my whole being dissolved into an ink blot, a fan of music or a multicoloured ray of light, and these waves, these forms, grew to an infinite distance and then quietly paled to become unrecognizable. Oh, if all this had been possible, then I would have attained all my desires. Gradually I was overcome by feelings of fatigue and stiffness. It was a pleasant lassitude, as though gentle waves were radiating from my body. Then I felt that my life was starting to run backwards. One after another, I saw experiences from long ago. Events and situations of former days, pale and forgotten memories of my childhood – I did not merely see them, but I took part in them, actively feeling them. From one moment to the next I became younger and even more childlike. Then suddenly everything became indistinct and dark, and it seemed as though my whole being was hanging by a thin hook at the bottom of a deep dark pit. Then I broke off the hook and fell and fell, and there was no resistance to break my fall – it was a bottomless abyss, down to the inner core of an eternal night. Then, slowly, a long series of vague, indistinct images passed before my eyes. After this, I sank into complete oblivion."[23]

The first thing which strikes us in this description of the effects produced by opium is that there are a number of phenomena which also appeared in the descriptions of the effects of LSD and, to a lesser extent, of cannabis. As we shall elucidate below, many passages in S. Hedayat's description reveal a partial separation of the ethereal body from the physical body, and of the astral body from the physical and ethereal body. These effects were described in detail in the chapters on LSD and marijuana/hashish, and we can therefore deal with this more briefly below.

The effect of opium on the ethereal body

Before using opium, S. Hedayat expresses the hope: "... only the delicate smoke of opium could bring my thoughts together and grant me peace." This is actually what happens: "The state I had waited for came to me even more strongly than I had hoped: slowly my thoughts assumed great clarity and a delicate purity."

This is a beautiful description of the effects of opium on a person's ethereal body, particularly on that part of the ethereal body which became separated in the course of childhood development – at approximately the age of seven – from the structural and formative activity in the physical body. It then became available for the structural development and formation of thought processes – at about the age of seven the forces of growth and formative forces are partly converted into cognitive forces.[24] Rudolf Steiner expressed this as follows: "Man's thinking powers are the sophisticated powers which create form and growth."[25] Hedayat perceived the clear, pure, formative qualities of these thinking forces, these free ethereal forces, without any opacity caused by the worries, cares and memories of daily life ... "so that this miracle-producing drug would remove all the obstacles and veils from my eyes and drive out all the distant, towering and ashen memories which piled up in front of me."

This indicates that, in the first instance, opium influences the functions of the ethereal body and gradually – and partially – separates it from the physical body, with the result that the part of the ethereal body which is already free (the thinking forces) is the first to be perceived and experienced by the user's consciousness (astral body and Self). Subsequently, a non-lethal quantity of poison (cf. LSD) will increasingly raise part of the ethereal body above the physical body, so that it becomes possible for the ethereal forces which have become separated (incorporating the astral body and the Self) to float up and away with the free thinking forces as they "fly out": "It seemed to me that the law of gravity no longer applied to me, and I could fly freely after my thoughts, which were rich, wide-ranging and absolutely clear."

The ethereal body also becomes partly separated in the central area, in the rhythmic system: "Then it was as though a great weight had been removed from my chest. I was freed from the burden of my body. My whole being felt as though it had been assimilated into the silently growing world of plants in a tranquil form of existence which was yet full of enchanting, lovely forms and colours."

This experience of the ethereal world of plants is extremely interesting and fascinating, and Rudolf Steiner explained that "the ethereal plant is contained in man's lungs (middle area), and this ethereal plant grows from the lungs rather like a physical plant grows from the earth."[26] The user perceives these (plant-like) ethereal forces which are released from the lungs, and the free part of his ethereal body – his thinking forces – become combined with this: "The interrelationship between my thoughts disappeared, and they combined with their forms and colours. I was submerged in waves of the softest tenderness." Thus the ethereal body is partly separated from the lungs, which is also expressed in a slowing down of the respiration which takes places when opium is used. (In the case of an overdose, death results because the user stops breathing.)

The user's astral body and Self also perceive other effects on his own ethereal body as a result of the fusion of the released ethereal forces with it (see Chapter 4, LSD): "I could feel the beating of my heart and my pulse. All of this was full of the deepest significance, and at the same time filled me with an infinite sense of wonder." The process continues. The released ethereal forces, with the astral body and Self incorporated in them, are assimilated in the surrounding world and dissolve with the universe: "When my whole being dissolved into an ink blot, a fan of music or a multicolored ray of light, and these waves, these forms, grew to an infinite distance and then quietly paled to become unrecognizable."

To summarize, it is clear that one of the aspects of the effect of opium is that the user partly dies, just as we described with the effect of LSD. This means that it raises part of her ethereal body from the physical body, so that the ethereal forces which are released can dissolve in the surrounding universe. For the same reason it is to be expected that other experiences, which accompany the experience of partial death, will also occur such as the experience of looking back on all or part of a past life, and the experience of changing dimensions of time and space.

To begin with the first point, S. Hedayat wrote: "Then I felt that my life was starting to run backwards. One after another, I saw experiences from long ago. Events and situations of former days, pale and forgotten memories of my childhood – I did not merely see them, but I took part in them, actively feeling them. From one moment to the next I became younger and even more childlike." The famous English poet and author, Thomas De Quincey, an opium addict, had similar experiences. In his book, *Confessions of an English Opium Eater* (1822), he wrote: "Some of the most insignificant experiences from my childhood, or long-forgotten scenes from later years, often rose up, coming back to life. I am quite convinced that the memory actually cannot forget."[27] We will return later in this chapter to this aspect of the tremendous increase in the capacity to remember which is brought about by opium.

With regard to the changes in the experience of space and time caused by the partial separation of the physical and ethereal body, Thomas De Quincey wrote: "Perceptions of space and time were both enormously stimulated. Buildings and landscapes appeared to me in such gigantic dimensions that the natural eye was unable to grasp them. Space expanded and reached an indescribable size. However, this did not worry me as much as the tremendous expansion of time. Sometimes it seemed as though I had lived for seventy or a hundred years in a single night. Yes, sometimes I had the feeling as though a thousand years had passed, or at any rate a length of time which far exceeds the limits of human experience."[28]

The question of which ethereal types are most involved in the process of separation from the physical body suggests that most probably this involves chemical ether which is connected with water, the liquid element (see LSD). Hedayat's descriptions indicate this: "I was submerged in waves of the softest tenderness ... It was a pleasant lassitude, as though gentle waves were radiating from my body ... and these waves, these forms grew to an infinite distance ..." Thus these are the movements of waves as well as growing movements (ethereal forces are growth forces). This element of growth is also found in De Quincey: "Space expanded and achieved indescribable dimensions ... the tremendous expansion of time."

These chemical, ethereal forces (of growth) connected with water, the liquid element, are centred in the liver. Victor Bott wrote: "The liver is the centre of the "water organism", the conductor of our ethereal body."[29] Thus the ethereal forces are separated in the liver, and eventually this can result in an ethereal effect on the liver, and later possibly also in a physical effect. This is expressed, on the one hand, in the disruption of the metabolic processes and the process for maintaining body heat (building processes) and on the other hand, in a paralysis of the will, melancholy, depression and fear of life. (In anthroposophic medicine the liver is seen as the centre of the processes of growth and metabolism in the physical body – as the centre of vegetative life and as the centrally located source of heat, the "furnace" of the physical body. In addition, the liver is the centrally located point of contact for the will. In the case of slight organic damage and injuries, a person is no longer aware of the forces which build up life, and can therefore become melancholy, depressed and fearful of life, while the will and the drive to act declines or even becomes paralysed.)

This is a description of the effect of opium on the user's ethereal body. It should be remembered that ethereal forces are also separated in the lungs, resulting in a liberating, relaxed, and peaceful feeling, free of tension.

The effect of opium on the astral body

Soon after the opium started to work, Hedayat fell into "a state which was half-sleep and half-impotence ... slowly my thoughts assumed great clarity and a delicate purity". This reveals that his astral body had partly withdrawn from his physical and ethereal body (see Chapter 5, Marijuana/hashish), so that he fell into this dreamlike state of consciousness. Thomas De Quincey had similar experiences, and indicated that as a result of the effects of opium, dreams and reality increasingly intermingled, until they eventually fused to become one. That is why Schmidbauer and Vom Scheidt concluded in their *Handbuch der Rauschdrogen*: (Handbook of Hallucinogenic Drugs) "The opium smoker falls into a twilight state between sleep and waking. Dream images rise up even when consciousness is not entirely lost."[30]

Thus these are dream images. We should remember that all the experiences described up to now which are caused by the partial separation of the ethereal body from the physical body, as well as the experiences discussed below (e.g. see "The effect of opium on the Self" p. 139), take place wholly or partly in the dreamlike state of consciousness.

The separation of the astral body from the ethereal and physical body has a number of other consequences:

– As a result of the withdrawal of her astral body from certain parts of the nervous system, the user becomes anaesthetized, so that feelings of pain disappear. The *Handbuch der Rauschdrogen* describes this: "According to new research, opiates affect the organism as follows: apparently there are certain receptors in the brain which prefer to assimilate the toxin, which is actually an alien substance in the body. The concentration of opiates in these opiate receptors was particularly noticeable in the limbic system which is wrapped around the brain stem rather like a hem of tissue. This is where the amygdaloid bodies are found, an area of the brain which plays a role in reactions of fear and flight ... In general, it could be said that the opiate receptors[31] are found in areas of the brain which contain paths for conducting pain stimuli. This explains the painkilling effect of opiates."[32,33] Thus the astral body is wholly or largely driven out of the nervous system, so that the perception of feelings of pain or fear caused by the physical body do not penetrate consciousness, or do so to a much lesser extent. This applies to an even greater extent for pure morphine, as we shall see below.

– The partially separated astral body is able to connect much more than usual with certain parts of the nervous system of the spinal cord system,[34] so that it is possible for the user to perceive things which are normally concealed under the threshold of ordinary consciousness, viz., the wisdom which fills the whole world and which makes all of creation into one (see Chapter 5, Marijuana/hashish). Hedayat wrote: "The interrelationship between my thoughts disappeared and they combined with their forms and colours. I was submerged in waves of the softest tenderness. I could feel the beating of my heart and my pulse. All of this was full of the deepest significance ..."

It is the "night side" of consciousness which is experienced: the user sinks into a world of cosmic wisdom which cannot be perceived by normal (daytime) consciousness. This fills her body and revives it and builds it up, particularly during sleep. Through the nerves of the spinal cord system it reaches her consciousness in a dreamlike state.

On the other hand, the partially separated astral body can, to a greater or lesser extent, dissolve in the cosmic astral world so that the experiences in this astral world can reach consciousness in a dreamlike way (see Chapter 5, Marijuana/hashish).

In order to conclude the description of the effects of opiates on the astral body, we will refer in detail to the way in which Rudolf Steiner described the effects of opium on the astral body in one of his lectures.

"With regard to opium, it has an extremely strong effect on the astral body in the sense that it separates man from his physical body. When he is separated from his physical body he experiences this as a great feeling of well-being. For a while he is rid of his physical body, and this gives him a sense of well-being.

"It is so easy to say – and I am sure you have often heard it said – that sleep is a wonderful thing. However, with regard to sleep, man actually does not experience this wonderful state, precisely because he is asleep! He cannot directly experience this wonderful condition, but can merely get a 'taste' of it. Because he has had the 'taste', he often suggests that sleep is so wonderful. When someone takes opium, the juice of the poppy, he does become aware of this wonderful state because he is in his body as though he is asleep and awake at the same time".[35] (see Chapter 5, p.109)

Finally, the opium user becomes tired. Hedayat wrote: "Gradually I was overcome by feelings of fatigue and stiffness. It was a pleasant lassitude, as though gentle waves were radiating from my body." This tiredness is an expression of the fact that the astral body wishes to break away from the physical and ethereal body, so that it can then dissolve in the cosmic astral world, while on the other hand, it partly connects with the nervous system of the spinal cord. After Hedayat's intense experience of his past life, "suddenly everything became indistinct and dark". This is followed by his beautiful description of the process when his astral body and Self depart: "And it seemed as though my whole being was hanging by a thin hook at the bottom of a deep dark pit. Then I broke off the hook and fell and fell, and there was no resistance to break my fall – it was a bottomless abyss down to the inner core of an eternal night". It is a beautiful description because the astral body floating upwards and away into the virtually infinitely astral world is experienced by the Self which is connected to it in the mirror of the physical and ethereal body, so that the astral body and the Self which are actually floating upwards, seem to be falling "into a bottomless abyss", and to the conscious eye, seem to be crashing down . This can be illustrated by placing a mirror on the ground and then moving the hand up from its surface; it looks as though it is disappearing into the depths, falling down into the surface of the mirror.

However, this disappearance, this "dissolving" of the astral body and the Self in the astral and spiritual world can be accompanied by extremely unpleasant feelings. Daily consciousness is not prepared for the experience of sinking into the night, the experience of disappearance, the dissolving of the astral body and the Self in virtually endless depths – actually the heights – of the astral and spiritual worlds. Thomas De Quincey wrote: "Night after night I seemed to sink down into depths and sunless abysses – not metaphorically, but literally – into depths below depths, without any hope of rising up. When I woke up I often had the feeling that I had risen up. Nevertheless, I do not want to dwell on this, because there are no words for the darkness which follows the wonderful scenes, and which ultimately congeals into a darkness of suicidal despair".[36]

In the end, Hedayat fell asleep: "Slowly a long series of vague, indistinct images passed before my eyes. After this, I sank into complete oblivion ..." This means that just before losing consciousness, Hedayat momentarily experienced the quality of his astral body dissolving in the astral world, i.e. oblivion. In *The Science of the Secrets of the Soul*, Rudolf Steiner wrote: "What death is to the physical body and sleep is to the ethereal body, oblivion is to the astral body".[37] Like every other opium addict, this is what Hedayat wanted: to forget. He wrote: "... so that this miracle-producing drug would ... drive out all the towering, distant and ashen memories ... I wanted to surrender completely to this sleep of oblivion. ... Oh, if only this total oblivion were possible, if only it could be permanent ... "

To summarize what was discussed above, it may be said that because of the partial departure of the astral body from the physical and ethereal body, the opium user enters a dreamlike state in which the "towering, distant and ashen memories" in the ethereal body (memory) can no longer penetrate the astral body (consciousness) in the usual way.[38] The user has forgotten this; her partially separated astral body no longer perceives the everyday content of the memory in the ethereal body; all her anxieties, fears, problems and so on, have been banished from consciousness.

Finally, the user falls asleep: her astral body, and therefore her consciousness, now completely withdraws from the normal connection with the physical and ethereal body in the waking state (with the exception of the nerves of the spinal cord), and dissolves in the cosmic astral world. The user's last experience is of her consciousness (astral body) sinking away and disappearing into sleep.

The effect of opium on the Self

Paradoxically, Hedayat also enjoys the memory: "Then I felt that my life was starting to run backwards. One after another I saw experiences from long ago. Events and situations of former days – I did not merely see them, but I took part in them, actively feeling them. From one moment to the next I became younger and even more childlike."

We came across this experience of the enormous increase in memories in the discussion of the effect of opium on the user's ethereal body. It was explained how this was caused by the partial separation of the physical and ethereal body caused by the drug.

However, there is another possible cause. It seems probable that, as a result of the effect of the drug, the Self is also partially separated from its connection with the autonomic nervous system. When this happens, the result is that "the Self can make use of those connecting channels with the world which allow him to see all sorts of things in space and time from a distance, which are normally embedded in the Self, in the autonomic nervous system, so that these processes cannot be perceived".[39] Consequently it is possible for the Self to review vast areas of space and time (also see De Quincey's description, page 134).

As regards time, Rudolf Steiner wrote about the use of opium in Asia: "This Malaysian with his habitual use of opium, encounters something tremendous. He encounters the Self. What does this lead to? ... What enjoyment follows? He is delighted to find that his memory is awakened in a wonderful, tremendous way. He can rapidly review his whole life on earth and much more. On the one hand, this is terrible, because he achieves it by making his body sick; on the other hand, the desire to know the Self is so strong that he is unable to resist it". He also wrote: "When Turkish people use opium they declare they have been in paradise ... Malaysians use opium to achieve a state in which they discern an element of the eternal quality of the soul ... but unfortunately, when a person does this too much, it ruins him. When a person works too much, it ruins him; when a person thinks too much, it ruins him. And when a person constantly evokes excessively strong memories, this ruins his body."[40]

In this context Rudolf Steiner mentions the generally well-known symptoms of opium addiction, such as:
– a pale complexion;
– hollow eyes;

- weight loss; malfunction of the intestines and constipation;
- stiff rigid limbs; clumsy walking, inability to walk in a straight line;
- forgetfulness; disappearance of capacity to think logically;
- the whole body is undermined, and many die as a result.[40]

According to Rudolf Steiner, all these symptoms are the result of "excessively strong memories".[40] He also explained: "If man developed only memory, and everything which made an impression on him stayed in the memory, his ethereal body would have to bear more and more, and would become richer and richer. But at the same time, this would lead to inner desiccation."[41] Obviously this has a disastrous effect on the physical body.

To summarize: the Self is partially banished from the autonomic nervous system by the effect of opium, so that the user's memory becomes too strong, and at the same time undermines the physical body.

Because of the explosive increase in the memory – though not the everyday memory – while the user is under the influence of opium, she becomes particularly forgetful once the effect of the opium has worn off. It is as though her memory has been burnt up to such an extent that after a while she can no longer even remember how to place one foot in front of the other, i.e. how to walk normally. Finally, this enormous memory can burn up and destroy the mirror function of the brain which constitutes consciousness, and the addict dies as a result.[42]

Euphoria

As every opium addict knows, the departure of the ethereal body, astral body and Self from the physical body is accompanied by strong feelings of bliss and delight.[43] Rudolf Steiner wrote: "Being liberated (from these elements of the soul) is always associated with an increase in the spiritual elements. However, this is related to a sense of well-being and true pleasure, both directly and indirectly. What has been liberated, whether it is the ethereal body, the astral body or the Self, is in a sense dispersed in the spiritual world. This dispersal is wholly accompanied by inner feelings of bliss".[44]

By way of example, he refers in this context to the notes of a psychologically disturbed patient whose ethereal body, astral body and Self separated from the physical body from time to time. He wrote: "I waited for my attacks full of impatience .... I waited for the feelings of bliss ... I found that I could do everything easily; there were no obstacles of either a theoretical or practical nature. My memory suddenly achieved a rare degree of perfection ..."[45]

It is easy to imagine that these feelings of euphoria increase tremendously when opium is injected directly into a vein (in the form of a warm, watery opium solution, so-called O[pium] tincture), so that the opium reaches the internal organs and the brain via the bloodstream within a few seconds. The partial separation from the ethereal body, the astral body and the Self takes place with lightning speed; the elements of the soul "shoot out" of the physical body, and the accompanying sense of pleasure or euphoria takes place in an intense flash of bliss or pleasure. This applies to heroin to a greater extent as we shall see below.

The hangover

The opium user awakes from her swoon with a dreadful hangover, feelings of nausea, pain and restlessness, and often with a sense of guilt about what she has done, etc. In order to banish these feelings, she can obviously reach for the opium once again and if she does this repeatedly, she will become addicted.

The question arises why it is so painful to return to the body, to re-enter the physical and ethereal body with the astral body and the Self, to return to ordinary waking consciousness?

To understand this, it is necessary to briefly examine what happens during the process of awakening. In his short book, *Wesen und Sinn des Schmerzens* (The Essence and Sense of Pain), H. Hessenbruch described this process as follows: "When we wake up in the morning, this happens because our spiritual soul (astral body and Self) re-enters the body and actually "collides" with it. This can be visualized in very concrete terms. Admittedly, the extrasensory element does not have a spatial dimension, but when it comes into contact with the spatial body and penetrates it, there is a sort of collision. The extrasensory spiritual soul "collides" with the body when it wishes to re-enter it. The experience of this "collision" is the moment of awakening. This process, which takes place in a very concrete way upon awakening, means that the spiritual soul enters the physical body, encountering resistance in a sort of collision. However, as it compresses back into the body, following the initial resistance, this body becomes transparent and the spiritual soul can penetrate it".[46]

However, if the body has been poisoned by opium and is in disorder and broken to some extent, the astral body will not be able to intermingle with the physical body easily, as it does normally, because of the disharmony between the physical body undermined by the opium, on the one hand, and the returning astral body and Self of the user, on the other."[46]

Hessenbruch wrote: "The experience of this disharmony is pain ... With regard to other forms of pain such as headache, stomach ache, aching joints and so on, the experience is always one of disharmony, of some sort of disruption of the harmonious establishment and interaction of things and processes. In medicine, this is known as a disfunction of the organs ... Wherever we look, we will always find that physical pain is based on the experience of a process of tearing away, separation, disruption and destruction, a process of disharmony."[47]

This also applies to the hangover caused by opium: " The user's astral self returns to an alien physical body, as the result of the effect of opium, and the user experiences this disharmony, this inability to enter the changed physical body, as pain.[48]

An additional aspect is that, as a result of the drug, the astral body and the Self have been cast out of the physical and ethereal body rather violently so that, upon their return, the collision of these two elements of the soul with the physical body will be all the stronger (this is comparable to the movement of a pendulum: the higher the pendulum swings, the more powerful the downward movement). Thus, upon awakening, the astral body and the Self will collide with the physical body all the more powerfully. It is as though they crash into it, trying to penetrate at all costs, and the user will experience the disharmony which arises between the alienated physical body on the one hand, and the astral body and the self on the other hand, all the more strongly which means more painfully. As Olav Koob wrote in his book, *Drogensprechstunde* (Consultations about Drugs): "The further one goes out of the body, the more deeply one crashes back into it. This means that the soul connects with the physical body more intensely, causing pain to the body and soul."[49]

Withdrawal symptoms

A common symptom accompanying the regular use of opium as a drug is that to some extent the human organism becomes habituated and an increased dose is necessary – up to a certain toxic level – to achieve the desired effect, i.e. to drive the ethereal body (partially) and the astral body and Self (wholly or partially) out of the physical body. In other words, the user develops a tolerance (see Introduction). Moreover, when the regular or chronic use stops – and the supply of opium stagnates – this results in so-called "withdrawal" (abstinence) symptoms such as stomach cramps, muscular cramps, pain all over the body, restlessness and so on. These withdrawal symptoms disappear as soon as the drug is taken again, or when the user has managed to survive the withdrawal symptoms.

The question arises as to why these withdrawal symptoms appear and why they are so strong. In conjunction with what was said above, it may be said that because of the effect of opium, the ethereal body is (partially), and the astral body and the Self are (partially or wholly) driven out of the physical body which is permeated with the opium substance resulting in the opium trance. As long as there is a sufficient amount of opium in the physical body, then the ethereal body, the astral body and the Self cannot return, and the dreamlike state continues. However, as soon as the opium level (the alkaloid level) has fallen below a certain minimum in the blood and the tissues, as a result of metabolic processes, excretory processes and so on, the ethereal body, the astral body and the Self "fall back" into the physical body, colliding with it powerfully and trying at all costs to penetrate, resulting in the violent pain of the waking state: withdrawal.

However, when the physical body becomes more and more alienated and habituated to the metabolism of the opium after repeated use, as in the case of addiction,[50] the physical body becomes increasingly impenetrable, "denser" for the addict's astral body and Self. The disharmony between the physical body on the one hand and the astral body and the Self on the other hand increases. As a result, the battle of the astral body and the Self to re-enter the physical body and "repossess" it becomes even more vehement. This means that the withdrawal symptoms become more painful and there may be severe cramps.

Hessenbruch wrote: "When the spiritual soul enters the body but cannot penetrate it, this results in what is generally known in medicine as 'cramps' ... Cramps are always a sign that the extrasensory aspect of man is trying to penetrate the body with his spiritual soul in some way, but is unable to do so ... All cramps are the expression of the fact that the healthy, normal flow of spiritual matter cannot take place, but that it 'becomes stuck'. This is also what causes the pain."[51]

Thus we see that the marked upward movement of the astral body and the Self, and the powerful downward, falling movement of these two elements of the soul into the distorted, compacted, alienated, physical body lead to the symptoms and experiences of severe muscular pains and painful cramps, etc.[52] As described above, this is like the pendulum of a clock: the upward movement of the astral body and the Self (i.e. the movement of separation, expansion and dissolving), and all the physical consequences, such as lower blood pressure and slowing down of the respiration, are followed by the downward movement of these two elements of the soul (i.e. the compacting movement of re-entry) which results, for example, in raised blood pressure and accelerated respiration.

To illustrate this, we will end with an extract from J.H. van Epen: "It is noticeable that, in general, the symptoms of abstinence are the opposite of the symptoms which appear while the user is under the influence of the drug. By way of example[53], someone who regularly uses opium, morphine or heroin is calm, with constricted pupils, slow intestinal functions (obstipation) and inhibited sexual functions. During withdrawal the user is restless, with dilated pupils, rapid intestinal functioning with stomach cramps and diarrhoea, and an uninhibited sexual functioning, exhibited, for example, in the form of spontaneous ejaculations and orgasms (which are usually experienced as being unpleasant)"[54]

This brings us to the conclusion of the discussion of the effect of opium on the different elements of the human organism. We saw that opium has a strong effect on three of these elements (the ethereal body, the astral body and the Self) through the physical body, which explains why this drug changes consciousness so effectively.

In conclusion, I refer those who would like to see the description given above in a broader perspective (in relation to spiritual science), to footnote 55. This may shed some light on some of the phenomena which are also closely related to the effect of opium, viz. the unearthly "paradise-like" atmosphere which the user enters, and the paradox of oblivion and memory, which is also the result of the use of opium.[55]

The effects of morphine

William Burroughs wrote: "You first feel morphine at the back of your legs, then at the back of your neck, and then a wave of relaxation spreads through the body so that your muscles are slack on your bones, and you seem to be floating without any boundaries, as though you are lying in warm salt water. When this wave of relaxation passed through the tissues of my body ..."[56]

Just before injecting himself, Hans Fallada wrote: "... just a very short moment, and then a solemn peace will flow through my limbs."[57] He continued: "I felt the tingling in my body and the wonderful secret sliding warmth. There are a thousand thoughts in me, because my brain is strong and free."[58]

Following an intravenous injection, René Stoute wrote: "All the pain disappeared from my body, a warm feeling spread gently through my veins and the tension disappeared ...". A little later, he continued: "The morphine was like a comfortable base in my stomach ...".[59]

In other words, morphine results in warmth, relaxation and the disappearance of pain.

An examination follows below of the effect of this drug on the various elements of the human organism in terms of the three different organic systems: the metabolic system, rhythmic system, and nervous, sensory system, including the brain.

The metabolic system

This also includes the limbs, as the muscles, particularly those of the limbs, play a major role in the metabolic and digestive processes of the human organism.[60] The muscles relax, which means that the astral body – which is always responsible for tension, alertness, activity and movement – withdraws from it; it is as though the muscles fall asleep and the user experiences this as a flow or wave of relaxation passing through her limbs and muscles.

It is a warm wave, which indicates that the ethereal forces, particularly the forces of ethereal heat, partly separate from the metabolic processes involving heat, particularly in the gastric area with the centre of the liver. As a result, the user experiences inner warmth, though externally she cools down in physical terms. In this context, Van Epen wrote: "Morphine and heroin users have a slightly lower body temperature than people who do not use these substances."[61]

We can also look at this from another perspective, in the sense that forces of ethereal heat are also released in the heart and circulatory system – the real organism where heat is generated in humans – as a result of the effect of morphine. Consequently the user experiences the pleasant ethereal heat.

As regards the metabolic system, morphine and heroin also have the following effects:[62]

"– a reduction in the movements of the intestines (peristalsis) resulting in constipation;
– an inhibition of sexual function, a loss of interest in sexuality,

frequently leading to impotence in men and the absence of menstruation in women;
- a reduction in urine production;
- a reduction in particular hormone levels in the body, including corticosteroids or adrenocorticotropic hormones."

These symptoms reveal that the astral body withdraws from all these organs to a great extent; they lose their tension, their activity, their mobility: the physical basis of the user's will is more or less rendered inactive. However, this does not occur without a battle; for example, the involuntary smooth muscular tissue of the pyloric sphincter, gall bladder, bile ducts, and sphincter, which are caused by the attempts of the astral body to penetrate these areas.[63] However, the separation and the sense of tranquillity is the dominant feeling: "Life is beautiful, it is so sweet and a wave of happiness rolls through my limbs; all sorts of small nerves move about like delicate water plants in a clear pond. I saw rose leaves." (This was Hans Fallada's description after an injection of morphine.)[64]

The rhythmic system

In this area morphine also separates the astral body (wholly or partly) from its connection with the physical and ethereal body. Morphine and heroin slow down breathing and inhibit the function of the heart.[65] This state of reduced activity is characteristic of the way these organs function during sleep, when the astral body is separated from the normal connection with the physical and ethereal body in the waking state. The stimuli which cause coughing are also inhibited. In the case of serious poisoning, the ethereal body is also separated from its connection with the physical body, which can result in death: "In the case of a heroin or morphine overdose the breathing becomes extremely slow... If the breathing stops when an overdose is taken, this results in death, unless action is taken quickly, for example, with artificial respiration or by administering an antidote, an 'antagonist'."[66]

The sensory nervous system

As we described for the effect of opium, morphine (and heroin) draws the astral body from that part of the nervous system and the brain which is responsible for conducting impulses of pain amongst other things (see p. 136). Van Epen wrote: "The effect of morphine and heroin is to inhibit the functions of the central nervous system, and of the brain ..."[66] This is why morphine and heroin are such unparalleled painkillers, and why the effect of morphine lasts longer than that of heroin, as described above.

To summarize, it may be said that morphine actually anaesthetizes the user, resulting in a more or less vegetable existence, by removing her astral body wholly or partly from the three systems of organs. As a result, she enters a blissful, warm, soft, light, dreamy and sleepy state of consciousness. "Morphine is a quiet, tender joy, white and flowery, and it makes its disciples happy." This is how the writer and morphine addict, Hans Fallada, described this drug.[67] René Stoute described it as follows: "Saturated with morphine, I dozed off in my chair, escaping time (illusion, illusion), the contours became vague, unpleasant thoughts evaporated, sins ceased to exist, there was no karma, there were no gnawing pains, there was no boredom and my consciousness became paralysed in a weightless void. My heavy eyelids closed. Sleep is where no trespasser can enter, it dances on soft slippers and in warm colours. Sleep does not judge, and helps you to forget. You do not have to do anything, you do not have to want anything: no thoughts, feelings, nothing more... nothing. This is what morphine can do for you."[68]

No cares, no sins, no karma, no judgement, no memories, no thoughts, no feelings, no will ... no Self!

The Self rises up from the body and the soul on the wings of ethereal heat. This is released by the circulatory system, which penetrates all three systems of organs.[69] It then becomes separate in a paradise of being alone... with itself. Hans Fallada wrote: "I am all alone in the world, I have no obligations, all is vanity and only pleasure matters".[58] He continued: "I am everywhere, I am everything, I alone am the world and God. I do and I forget, and everything passes."[70] René Stoute described morphine addicts in the following terms: "Pure morphine addicts and heroin addicts wished for a constant state of anaesthesia and long hours of sleep. They woke up only to go back to sleep as soon as possible. They lived side by side and did things together, but always remained by themselves. All alone."[71] Alone with morphine, their beloved morphine.

Hans Fallada wrote: "I think of you, my sweet girl, whom I lost a long time ago. Now my only love is morphine. She is bad, she tortures me immeasurably, but she also rewards me in a way you cannot imagine. This love is truly in me. She fills my intellect with a clear light, and by her light I see that all is vanity and that I live only to enjoy this pleasure ..." "Penetrate more deeply, my dear friend, and bring me to even greater ecstasy ... " "And I am full of bliss and know that I am alone with her and that nothing else matters." "But then I suddenly realize that the effect of the morphine has worn off! My body is shaking again. Abandoned by my beloved, I have not even managed to get another prescription."[72]

The effects of heroin

This condition of extreme isolation is even stronger in heroin; the user enters her own warm cosmos where she is alone with herself. The Self has lost virtually all the connections with her own body, soul and with other people; fears, worries and pain no longer get to her; she is "closed" to herself and to the world. This isolation is clearly expressed in a poem by Jenny G, aged 19:

Dear little sister

Dear little sister,
You princess on a pea,
Most treasured queen,
I love you,
And only you,
You give me independence
You render me insensitive to pain and sorrow.
– What do I have to do with other people?

Your warmth penetrates me,
Completely surrounds me.
In your waves I feel completely protected,
Against cold and steel arrows,
Clad in a skin,
Thin, elastic and tough like that of the egg.
I float on your waves,
Towards that
Which I ardently desire,
Towards the peace which only you can give me.

In my veins your fire blazes,
Glows in my innards,
Without burning them.
My constricted soul relaxes,
Satisfies the desires of my heart.
On your wings,

> I slide into the abyss
> Of my spirit, of your spirit,
> With music in the background ...[73]

The forces of ethereal heat which have been released penetrate and surround the user's inner being; inside the outwardly thick, cold membrane it is beautifully warm.

But heroin does more than this: on the wings of ethereal heat the user's Self flies on to the free part of the ethereal body, to that part of the ethereal body which surrounds the head area in the widest sense, and which is responsible for cognitive processes. The user becomes all "head". Because of the partial separation of her astral body, she has become insensitive and closed to everyday pains, fears and cares which arise in the body and in the soul. It is as though her consciousness has withdrawn into the "top of a lighthouse". A few examples are given below:

— "It is as though my head is cut off from the rest of my body, I am completely in the here and now."[74]
— "Heroin makes you cool and calculating and protects you against fear."[75]
— "I felt raised up above myself, standing far above myself and everything else. I was cool. In a sense my Self, my physical Self, was down there, very small, below me, like a person seen from an airplane. At that moment it did not really matter to me if that other Self fell flat on his face or not."[76]
— Olaf Koob described the effect as follows: "This substance turned the person into someone who was all 'head' ..., with an icy consciousness and seemingly rigid and adapted to the outside world. Heroin divides the soul from the intellect, and therefore has a property which explains why it is taken by young people today: it drives out fear. Adapting by removing fear – is it possible to conceive of a better and more effective temptation nowadays?"[77]

To summarize it may be said that:
— Heroin partly raises the ethereal body from the physical body, so that the forces of ethereal heat are released in addition to the ethereal forces from the lungs (see morphine). – Heroin also wholly or partly raises the astral body from the physical and ethereal body, resulting in the anaesthetic, painkilling and tranquillizing effect.

- Heroin helps the Self to break away from its connection with the other elements of the soul, on the wings of ethereal heat.
- Heroin does allow a connection between the Self and the free part of the ethereal body so that the Self, isolated from the body and soul can continue to think in a cold, distant and instrumental way, devoid of the warmth of the soul and heart, until the wholly separated astral body eventually takes the Self with it into the world of unconsciousness, the world of sleep.

It is easy to imagine that the euphoria accompanying these processes of separation will be very great, particularly when the heroin is injected directly into the blood so that it reaches the internal organs and the brain within a few seconds. A few examples are given below:
- "The flash arrived like a tidal wave against the dykes. A pleasant warmth glowed through my whole body."[78]
- "This feeling of nirvana is even more intense when heroin is injected (compared to morphine, and opium which is not as strong). For someone who hankers after drugs, nothing in the world could be more desirable than the flash of release, when the heroin enters the blood and is taken to the brain, where it erases the truly hellish pains of withdrawal at a single stroke."[79]
- "One difference with morphine is that heroin goes to the brain much more quickly because it passes through the cerebral membrane more easily and therefore produces a stronger flash than morphine."[80]

But the price is high. In the first place, the euphoria becomes a less and less important reason for using heroin, and is replaced by the fear of the withdrawal symptoms expected by the user: "Time is the great spoilsport. Time stands and waits on the threshold. Time will hold you responsible." These are the words of the addict/author, Arie Visser.[81] Van Epen expressed this as follows: "A four to six hour rhythm is imposed on the addict by the level of opiates in his blood. He never feels normal but is either stoned or ill. Eventually the normal rhythms of life (sleeping-waking, hunger-satisfaction of hunger, working-resting, sexual needs – satisfaction, and so on) are pushed completely to the background. Addicts never 'keep to our time', they always go by their own heroin-dictated time."[82]

In addition, the physical and psychological condition of the addict eventually deteriorates. Apart from the physical effects of using heroin which were described for morphine, there may be a number of other side effects, such as a grey complexion, defects of the lungs, liver and blood (lymphocyte abnormalities), attacks of angina pectoris, stomach and intestinal complaints, skin rashes, outbreaks of sweating following the slightest exertion, injuries to the nervous system, loss of teeth, damage to the sexual organs such as lowered levels of testosterone in the blood, a loss of potency in men and interrupted menstrual cycles in women. In addition, this physical deterioration is often accompanied by psychological problems. In the *Handbuch der Rauschdrogen* (Handbook of Hallucinatory Drugs), this is described as follows: "Initially, rational activity remains intact to a surprising degree, despite the disruption of perception caused by the drug. Despite many years of abusing opiates, intellectuals can continue to make important scientific and artistic contributions. However, the constant undermining of their powers of concentration, the loss of memory, and, finally, psychotic states eventually intervene in this area to such an extent that it often   results in secondary loss of intellect and 'stupidity'."[83]

Thus we see that as a result of the use of heroin, there is a general deterioration of the addict's physical and psychological condition. Many addicts are aware of this, but suppress the feeling by taking more heroin. Moreover, the fear of withdrawal symptoms, and of the emptiness and depression which follow this, prevent many people from ceasing to use the drug.

How are these withdrawal symptoms experienced by heroin addicts deprived of their drug? When William Burroughs kicked the habit in a police cell, he wrote: "I was lying on the narrow wooden bunk and turned from one side to the other. My body felt raw and swollen; flashes of pain shot through my flesh where the frozen state of addiction was thawing in a way that was torture. I turned on to my stomach and my legs slid off the bunk. I fell forwards and the rounded side of the bunk which had been polished smooth by the friction of clothes rubbed my crotch. There was a sudden flow of blood to the genitals when I made this contact. There was an explosion of sparks behind my eyes; my legs constricted with cramp – it was the orgasm of a hanged man when his neck is broken.

... My blood was thick and concentrated with the loss of fluid from my body. In the forty-eight hours that I had no heroin, I lost ten pounds in weight. It took the doctor twenty minutes to get enough blood for a blood test, because my thick blood constantly clotted in the needle ...

The third day and night of withdrawal are generally the worst.

After the third day the condition generally recedes. I felt a cold fire over the entire surface of my body as though my skin was covered with uninterrupted chicken pox. It was as though ants were crawling under my skin.

It is possible to separate yourself from most pain – injuries to the teeth, eyes and genitals give rise to special problems – so that the pain is experienced as a neutral stimulus, but it seems impossible to escape from the pain of withdrawal. It is the other side of the kick which heroin provides. The kick of junk is that you have to have the stuff. Junkies run on junk time and junk metabolism, they are subject to the junk climate. They warm up and cool down with junk. The kick of junk is life under junk conditions. You can no more escape from withdrawal than you can escape from the kick with a shot".[84]

In his book, *De drugs van de wereld, de wereld van de drugs* (The drugs of the world, the world of drugs), J.H. Van Epen summarized the symptoms as follows: "With opiates with a short half-life, such as morphine or heroin, the first withdrawal symptoms occur within a few hours after the last dose; they are strongest on the second or third day and slowly diminish in intensity in the course of the fourth to sixth day. After ceasing to take an opiate with a longer half-life like methadone, the symptoms arise only after a day; they are strongest after five to seven days and then gradually diminish in the course of one to three weeks. The withdrawal symptoms may vary from being virtually absent to extremely serious. In rare cases they may be life-threatening.

There are a number of factors which influence the nature and intensity of withdrawal symptoms. First, there is the severity and length of the addiction. People who have used heroin for only a short while generally experience mild withdrawal symptoms. Where large or very large quantities have been used, the symptoms are more serious. In addition, the patient's general physical condition is very important.

Withdrawal syndromes are usually more serious in people who are more seriously ill and in patients with a generally physically poor condition. The patient's psychological condition is also important: some scream blue murder, even though there are few objective signs of withdrawal, while others seem to tolerate severe withdrawal symptoms relatively easily ...

The symptoms of the opiate withdrawal syndrome are as follows: a fearful, restless and rather caved-in countenance, cold and clammy skin, large eyes with dilated pupils, a runny nose, hiccups, often constant yawning, a feeling of being alternately hot and cold, stomach cramps with a great deal of flatulence and diarrhoea, sometimes vomiting. Muscular pains and cramps in the back and legs. Gooseflesh, hair standing on end, increased intestinal movement, slightly raised pulse rate, blood pressure and body temperature. All this is usually accompanied by an unquenchable desire to take more opiates".[85]

An examination of these symptoms shows that the user's astral body and Self in particular are trying to re-enter the physical body from which they have become separated and which has become habituated to an opiate metabolism. As a result, there is a rise in pulse rate, blood pressure and body temperature, the metabolic organs start to move again and the ex-user wakes up.

And how! Because the astral body and the Self separated so strongly, these two elements of the soul re-enter the physical body with great downward force. In a sense they cause it to become over-conscious and over-awake (big eyes, hair standing on end), as though they are pressing it out: runny nose, watery eyes, a loss of body fluids. However, the physical body resists; it has lost its transparency for the astral body – particularly after long term use – and has become dense, hard and cold (William Burroughs: "Flashes of pain shot through my flesh where the frozen state of addiction was thawing in a way that was torture"). Therefore, the astral body and the Self are constantly rejected and bounce back with the result that the blood pressure and the body temperature fall. When the addict withdraws, he becomes slightly relaxed and constantly yawns.

Then the astral body and the Self re-enter with great force and this overactivity of the astral body causes more pain accompanied by cramps: the disharmony between the compact changed physical body and the above-mentioned higher elements of the soul has become so great that when the astral body and the Self repeatedly enter, this causes severe pain and cramps.

And so it goes on, up and down, for days and nights on end, often accompanied by panic attacks and depression until the astral body and the Self have re-established some form of harmony with the physical body and can re-enter it to some extent. However, it remains a difficult situation for a long time; the ex-addict is unstable, oversensitive, over-emotional, irritable and easily exhausted, and feels empty and depressed. In this context, Van Epen even talks of a post-detoxification syndrome which can last for many months.[86]

Nevertheless, in this respect is should be noted that the environment can play an important role in the withdrawal process, in the sense that the quality of the environment will influence the intensity of the withdrawal symptoms.

After all, the astral body and Self of the addict withdrawing from drugs are submerged in the astral and moral quality of the environment (colours, shapes, atmosphere and so on), while even the quality of the astral bodies and of the "Selves" of the people around her will influence the intensity of the withdrawal symptoms. Going through the process of withdrawal in a cold, indifferent and possibly hostile environment (for example, in a police cell), will therefore in most cases be much more painful and difficult than in a warm, caring, helpful and involved environment.

Here is another example. Roorda described that when these problems of addiction were still new and unknown, the process of withdrawal was much worse. This was because everyone was afraid of it. Not only the patients themselves, but also the medical profession and other staff in institutions. This anxiety was contagious, and because of the anxiety the symptoms were felt all the more strongly.[87] The astral body and the Self of the former addict are therefore influenced by the environment in which the withdrawal process takes place.

This brings us to the end of our description of the effects of heroin. In conclusion, it should be mentioned that the use of heroin entails great dangers for the survival of the addict. Under present circumstances, heroin is an illegal drug and consequently associated with the use of dirty needles, prostitution to finance the habit, poor quality of the drug and so on. A study in West Berlin revealed that the number of fatalities amongst male heroin addicts was twelve times as high as those of their contemporaries who were not addicts. For women, the mortality rate was twenty-nine times as high.[88] Furthermore, other follow-up studies revealed that at least 15% of a group of addicts can be expected to have died within ten years (fifteen years after starting to use heroin an average of only 35% of users had managed to stop).[89]

Methadone

To conclude this chapter on opiates, we will devote some attention to the synthetic substitute, methadone.

Methadone (Polamydon, Symoron) is a purely synthetic opiate.

It was first synthesized in Germany in 1940 without the use of any natural raw materials. Nowadays, methadone is used mainly as a substitute for heroin because it has to be taken only once every twenty-four hours. (For heroin, this is four to six times per twenty-four hours.) The result is that the addict is able to function with a much more normal rhythm of days and nights (instead of being concerned with the next shot of heroin all day). In addition, methadone has the advantage that it can be taken orally – either in the form of tablets – or in the form of a thick sugary syrup which cannot really be injected so that the dangers of intravenous injections (blood poisoning, inflammation of the veins, abscesses, liver infections, infection of the AIDS virus and so on caused by the use of dirty needles), do not apply.

Initially it was thought that methadone was the miracle cure which would not be addictive, while it would still have the same effect as heroin. However, these expectations were not realized. Methadone also resulted in physical addiction and proved to give rise to even longer and more difficult withdrawal symptoms than heroin, at least when the user stops taking the drug altogether from one day to the next.

As regards the effect of methadone, it produces a strong feeling of well-being just like opiates. Physically there are also great similarities to the effects of morphine and heroin (particularly persistent constipation, severe sweating and, in the case of a high dose, a lot of itching). Therefore, we refer to the description of the effects of opiates (particularly morphine and heroin) for the effects, the hangover, the withdrawal symptoms and so on.

Nevertheless, many methadone addicts also use heroin because they crave the more intense euphoria of the intravenous "flash". The hope that the daily use of methadone (on prescription) would put an end to the criminal activities of ex-heroin addicts also proved unfounded: criminality (thefts, break-ins, robberies and so on) fell in most cases by only about 10%.[90]

Nowadays, methadone is used in two different ways: on the one hand, in the form of a cure based on reduced dosages for heroin addicts who gradually withdraw from the drug. In this case the addict is prescribed a starting dosage of methadone which is reduced to zero in the course of a few weeks. On the other hand, it can also be taken regularly on prescription, so that the methadone addict continues to take the same amounts of methadone every day for years.

7

Alcohol

Alcohol is the most widely used hard drug in the world. In 1950, a study by the United Nations estimated the number of users at one billion, and the number of people addicted to alcohol at twenty million (cf. at that time the number of people using hashish/marijuana was estimated at 200 million).[1] Since then, there has been a marked increase in the use of alcohol. In the Netherlands, the number of people who drink a minimum of 8 glasses of alcohol per day rose from an estimated 124,000 in 1960 to approximately 760,000 in 1979[2], i.e. an increase by a factor of six. This was followed by a slight decline to approximately 664,000 in 1990.[2] Of these 664,000 people, about 186,000 drank on average more than 16 glasses of alcohol per day.[2] (Also see the graph on p.27.)

Here are some more figures:
— In 1950, 2 litres of pure alcohol was consumed per head of the population in the Netherlands;[3] in 1979, this was 9.1 litres, in 1990, 8.2 litres.[4]
— 40% of children between 12 and 14 drink alcohol occasionally and, from the age of 16, the pattern of consumption is the same as for adults.[a] An increasing number of women drink alcohol. Thirty years ago, the ratio between male and female alcoholics was 20 to 1; now it is 3 to 1.[5,b]
— The number of hospital admissions due to alcohol rose from 1,174 in 1969 to 4,177 in 1979. In 1990 there were 2,634 admissions for alcohol abuse.[6]
— The number of deaths where cirrhosis of the liver was the primary cause rose from 401 in 1960 to 745 in 1979, and to 781 in 1987.[7] With regard to cirrhosis of the liver as the secondary cause of death, these figures were: 123 in 1960, 420 in 1979, and 332 in 1987.[8,c]
— At the same time the revenue from the tax on alcoholic drinks rose from ƒ217,336,000 in 1960 to ƒ1,811,779,000 in 1991, an increase by a factor of eight.[9]

- In the mid-1970s, 25% of all crimes in the Netherlands were committed under the influence of alcohol. These were predominantly crimes of aggression.[10]
- In countries such as Canada and the United States, where the examination and recording of the use of alcohol are compulsory in the case of fatal car accidents, it was found that 40 to 50% of people who die on the roads had more than 0.8 per thousand parts of alcohol in the blood.[11] (In the Netherlands it is a crime to drive with more than 0.5 per thousand parts of alcohol.)
- In the United States, 40,000 people die every year as a result of alcohol abuse (cf. 4,000 people die as a result of heroin abuse).[12]
- In the former Federal Republic of Germany the social costs of alcoholism were estimated in 1989 to amount to 30 billion marks per year.[13]

To summarize, it may be said that alcohol is a dangerous drug. How has it come to be the most widely used hard drug in the world? What is the history of alcohol?

Alcohol in history

As we mentioned in the chapter on the history of the use of drugs, alcohol – in the form of wine – was described in the Old Testament when Noah planted a vineyard and became drunk from drinking wine (Genesis 9: 20–21), and when King Melchizedek "brought forth bread and wine, and he was the priest of the most high God" (Genesis 14:18).

Wine is the oldest alcoholic drink in the world. Together with grain and flax, the vine is one of the oldest crops cultivated by man. Wine was known to the ancient Sumerian-Babylonian-Egyptian civilization in about 3000 BC. Pictures of vineyards, the harvesting and preparation of wine dating from 2400 BC have been found in Egypt. In 2225 BC, King Hammurabi of Babylon passed the first law on drinking to regulate the use of alcohol. A few centuries later, beer also became widely used. As far as we know, the Sumerians were the first to brew beer. From there it also passed to Egypt.

However, in antiquity wine was the predominant drink. From the beginning, it was used above all to help people acquire a new consciousness. This was particularly true during the Greek civilization from approximately 700 BC, and manifested itself in the cult of Dionysus.

Rudolf Steiner described this cult as follows: "You know that the cult of Dionysus was related to wine... In the course of man's development alcohol had a mission to fulfil. No matter how strange it may sound, its mission was to prepare man's body in such a way that it was cut off from its relationship with the Divine, so that the individual 'I am' could emerge. Alcohol works by cutting man off from the spiritual world in which he operated before. In our own time, alcohol still has this effect. Alcohol has certainly served a purpose. In future, people will be able to say in the most literal sense that it was the task of alcohol to pull man down into the material world so far that he would become selfish, and that alcohol would lead him to demand the use of his self for his own purpose, so that it would no longer serve the whole nation ... Alcohol has removed man's capacity to feel at one with the universe in the higher worlds."[14]

This is in complete contrast with the effects of hashish and opium. Alcohol does not direct humankind upwards into the spiritual world, but downwards, to the earth. It severed the drinker's ties with the spiritual world, stimulated a feeling of independence from the world of the gods and gave him a sense of responsibility for his own acts and decisions.

However, this development was not without danger and therefore the mission of alcohol was couched in the Dionysus cult which evolved from the wisdom of the mysteries. What did this cult entail? And who was Dionysus?

According to the *Dionysiaka* by the Greek poet, Nonnos,[15] Dionysus was born from the union of Zeus and his mortal wife, Semele, after Semele's mother had lamented the sad fate of people on earth. Zeus was moved by her laments and decided to conceive Dionysus to send him and the vine to mankind for consolation. Despite his premature birth, and despite a great deal of opposition from the world of the gods, Dionysus grew up to become a fair youth who gave his love to the young satyr, Ampelos, with whom he engaged in competitions which he enjoyed enormously. One day, Ampelos was killed by a bull. Dionysus was overcome with grief. To console him, Zeus transformed the dead Ampelos into a vine, and at the same time showed Dionysus how to prepare wine, so that Dionysus and wine could start to fulfil their mission from that time.

First, Dionysus went east to India. But the people of the East were not interested in this new young god and remained loyal to their own gods. This led to conflict. On both sides the gods joined in to help, and after seven years the Indians were conquered. This is traditionally expressed in the belief that Dionysus brought agriculture, apiculture (honey), viniculture and science to the people of the East.

But he was not successful in the Arab countries. Dionysus had to flee and temporarily find shelter in the Red Sea. (Subsequently alcohol was forbidden by Islam.) Ultimately Dionysus conquered his opponents virtually everywhere. Most of the gods supported him, and even Apollo tolerated his presence; at several sites of the Mysteries, Dionysus and wine were even worshipped. In Delphi, Dionysus was actually worshipped with Apollo.

Many myths and stories about Dionysus – and wine – describe how his arrival saw the former cosmic projection of a dreamlike consciousness based on imagery make way for a much more individual, awake and intellectual consciousness. However, this also entailed the danger that people could become trapped by the confusion and disharmony which accompanied this transition. This is why Dionysus is often depicted in the company of a colourful troupe of followers wearing animal skins, while his retinue also included animals, bacchantes and satyrs – these are all images of the fact that the animal forces separated from cosmic harmony would henceforth be part of mankind's development. In this dangerous world the straight staff of Dionysus (the Thyrsos staff) served as a support for man so that he could defend himself- not by using it to strike, but by touching it – and which he could use to remain upright in this field of animal forces: this is an image for the strength of the Self.

But there was also the danger of selfish isolation and conflict, for man had been abandoned by divine guidance and had to learn to find his own way and build up new social structures with the help of his newly awoken intellectual capacities.

In the cult of Dionysus an attempt was made to counter these dangers by drinking wine in large quantities communally, so that people experienced a new sense of community, different from the ties of blood and the family. The people were taught to control themselves as much as possible – despite being under the influence of large amounts of wine – so that they could dominate the inner "animals". That is why the cult of Dionysus was a cult of celebration, an orgiastic cult in which animals were sacrificed communally, particularly the goat and the bull, as a symbol of man's inner "animal" forces which were being sacrificed. In addition, games were played to practice control of the body and soul with the Self. Simonis described one of these games: "A 'sack' filled with wine was fashioned from a goatskin turned inside out. It was smeared on the outside with olive oil so that it was slippery. Then, one by one, everyone at the feast tried to jump onto it on one leg and remain standing. Obviously this was done *after* drinking wine. It is easy to imagine the self-control required for this exercise. Anyone who fell off was mocked by the others, and whoever succeeded in staying on was hailed as being victorious."[16]

Self-control and a positive way of dealing with differences of opinion which arose were also practised in so-called "symposia" *after* drinking wine, where discussions were held about philosophical questions, or riddles were solved or all sorts of intellectual verbal tricks were performed.[17]

Thus all these activities were aimed at establishing the young Self in the body and soul, so that it was at home there, by following the path of self-control. The hangover experienced after drinking wine was very helpful in this respect. The pain, nausea etc. helped man to become more conscious of his own physical body, his own piece of earth, and this contributed to a stronger connection between the higher parts of his being (ethereal body, astral body and Self) and the physical body.

However, gradually the cult of Dionysus became decadent. The original intentions became increasingly lost in the background, The feasts lost their original sparkle, and at the time of the Roman Empire the large-scale use of alcohol was in danger of getting out of control in the cult of Bacchus. In 186 BC the Bacchanalia, the orgiastic cult festivities of Dionysus and Bacchus, were prohibited throughout Italy on penalty of death. This was because of the sexual orgies and murders which allegedly took place during the Bacchanalia. However, the prohibition of the Roman Senate did not prevent the ecstatic wine feasts from flourishing once again, after a while, so that they became increasingly integrated into Roman culture. It was at this time, when alcohol completely cut man off from the spiritual world on a large scale, appealing to the strongest selfishness in him, that Christ came to earth. Rudolf Steiner wrote: "At the same time that man was drawn down into the most profound selfishness by alcohol, the great strength emerged which could give man the impetus to reunite with the spiritual universe. On the one hand, man had to descend to the depths to become more independent; on the other hand, there was a great strength which could help to reveal the way back to the whole universe ..."

Dionysus is the splintered god which has penetrated individual souls so that the various elements of the soul no longer knew anything about each other. Alcohol, the symbol of Dionysus, splintered man into many pieces and surrendered him to the material world."[14]

In the first instance, Christ was in line with the Dionysus cult because he changed water into wine at the marriage feast of Cana (as an image for the ancient group consciousness of man which permeates everything and is dreamily submerged in the Divine world). Rudolf Steiner wrote: "In the first place Christ pointed out that the Self should become independent, and subsequently he turned to those people who had freed themselves from their blood relatives. He turned to the guests at the wedding where people were under the influence of alcohol ... .

It is as though the highest impulse descended to the customs of those times, because he expressed the greatest truth in the words and actions which suited the understanding of the people of the time. Thus, by means of a sort of Dionysus or sacrifice of wine Christ showed how man could be raised to Godliness. ... Christ went to the Galileans (Cana was in Galilee), who were not related by blood ... and carried out the first task in his mission. He conformed to their customs to such an extent that he changed the water into wine for them.

Let us remember what Christ really meant when he did this: he also wanted to bring a spiritual dimension to those people who had descended to the level of materialism symbolized by drinking wine."[14]

After this, Christ was able to fulfil his true mission which was described by Rudolf Steiner in the following words: "His mission consisted of bringing man the full power of the Self, the inner independence of the soul. Every individual Self should be able to feel completely independent and separate, and man shall be brought together with man through the love which is granted as a free gift ...

We should take careful note of Christ's words: my mission is such that it points to a very distant future; and people should be given a relationship with God as independent people, the love of God as a free gift of the independent Self."[14]

The mission related to alcohol described above is full of the coming of Christ as expressed by Rudolf Steiner: "Nowadays, when man is once again endeavouring to find the way back, and the Self has developed to such an extent that man can once again join together with divine and spiritual forces – now the time has come that a certain reaction is developing against alcohol, though initially this was still an unconscious reaction. This reaction has arisen because many people feel nowadays that something which once had a special meaning is not justified for all time."[14]

The Dionysus cult has come to an end; worshipping Dionysus as a God of the blood ties which will be broken, and of the instincts, passions and drives controlled by the Self, can make way for the inner acceptance of Christ as the bringer of the love of man for his fellow man, and of the free spiritual love of man for God. In this way Christ took the place of a vine. In the *Gospel According to St. John* he expressed this as follows: "I am the true vine", (John 15:1) and: "I am the vine stick and ye are the branches" (John 15:5). During the Last Supper his work culminated in this respect in changing His blood into wine. This completed the task of wine: wine has become the blood of Christ. To express the way the situation had changed, the Apostle Paul warned the first Christian believers against the traditional ways: "And be not drunk with wine, wherein is excess, but be filled with the Spirit." (Ephesians 5:18). A new way had opened.

In this respect it should not be forgotten that at the time when these events took place, viniculture and drinking wine were fairly standard practice in the vast Roman empire (which also included Palestine). For example, in many cities wine houses had been opened. These were houses where people drank wine together which they had brought along themselves. With the campaigns to Gaul and Germany, viniculture spread to the north and west of Europe. However, during the time of the Roman emperors, wine was greatly abused and eventually this contributed to the decadence and final downfall of the Roman Empire.

Another look at history shows that during the reign of Charlemagne (768–814), viniculture was encouraged and vineyards were planted from the Atlantic coast to northern Germany and northern Poland. However, most of these northern vineyards were lost in the course of time. The cold winters and imports of superior southern wines took their toll. In the end the areas around the Moselle and the Rhine in Germany and the areas around Bordeaux, the east of Paris (Champagne) and Burgundy produced the best wines. Even today excellent wines are produced there.

In about the 10th century there was a great change: the Arabs were the first to discover that the intoxicating substance in wine could be distilled and therefore concentrated. They called the "burning" wine (brandy) al-cohol which means the best and purest essence of a substance or "the spirit". This brandy which had a higher alcohol percentage than normal wine was mainly prescribed as a medicine in the Middle Ages, as were hashish and opium.

In the Middle Ages, beer, ale, cider and wine (particularly for the higher classes of society) were the most commonly used alcoholic drinks. They were drunk in taverns and other public places, but also in church. Aldo Legnaro described an English "church ale" as follows: "In Medieval England the 'church ale' was one of the regularly occurring occasions when people drank alcohol together ... This communal drunkenness had a sacred character and was an intoxicating experience of togetherness. This applied even more obviously to the 'glutton masses' which were held five times a year: the parish would gather together in church in the morning, everyone bought their own food and drink, attended mass and then celebrated at a feast which culminated with the total inebriation of all the participants (including the priest). Moreover, competitions were held between different parishes, for example to see who could eat most meat and drink most alcohol in honour of the Holy Virgin."[18] These celebrations very clearly corresponded to the ritual sacred feasts of the ancient Dionysus cult!

Another correspondence was that from time to time certain laws and prohibitions were introduced by the government to teach people to control themselves during these communal drinking events. For example, there was the commandment by the Anglo-Saxon King Edgar in the 10th century that all the barrels should be marked with standard signs. Anyone who drank more than this standard measure in one go was punished. However, during the Middle Ages drunkenness was not in itself considered in a negative light; it was accepted as man's third state of consciousness, next to sleeping and waking, provided the drunkenness remained within the rules prescribed from above. Within these rules people could drink unrestrainedly without fear of sanctions and without feeling ashamed.[19] However, for anyone who went beyond the permitted boundaries, for example by drinking constantly or at other times than during the ritual occasions, there were social controls which banished them from society. There is a poem dating from the first half of the 13th century about a stubborn drinker who first praised his master – wine – and drunkenness, and then tried to persuade the poet to do the same. This poem is as follows:

> I would ignore
> Your advice and your ideas
> Damned be your honour! ...

I would like
To leave you and wine together;
I will not take any notice of you henceforth!
And thus they parted.[20]

This was a serious sanction, because the consciousness of medieval man did not have such an individual character as it does now. In the Middle Ages people were more childlike and did not have the same sharply outlined personality structure. They had much more of a sense of being part of a larger whole. The attention was focused on the sum of the individual parts and not on individual, but on general, traits. "Individuum est ineffabile (The individual is unpronounceable). This statement by a medieval philosopher expresses the general approach of the time."[21] Therefore being rejected by society was an extremely serious sanction.

To summarize, it may be said that the use of wine and drunkenness in the Middle Ages was still closely related to the traditions of the ancient Dionysus cult. It was possible to become drunk communally with no feelings of shame or guilt as long as the social norms imposed by higher authorities were observed and provided that one had the inner control to keep to the prescribed norms and occasions. Anyone who broke the rules was punished by being cast out.

At the end of the 15th and the beginning of the 16th century a new period started in the history of European culture. The emergence of rationality and the development of scientific ideas increasingly required an active inner individual self-control. The control of the emotions and of one's own actions acquired primary importance. Self-control was raised to an art form. Baltasar Gracian (1601 – 1658), a Spanish Jesuit and moralist, formulated this more than a century later in the following words: "There is no greater dominion than that of a person over himself and over his feelings; this becomes a triumph of the free will."[22]

By this time drunkenness was viewed in a much more negative light. It was seen as a lack of self-control and as an obstacle to rational consciousness. In the 16th century the world became a more sober place; the ideal was one of "sober courage", i.e. a way of life which avoided extremes and was temperate in enjoyment. This also applied to the consumption of alcohol – moderation and controlled drinking were encouraged. The first temperance society (not an entirely teetotal society), the order of Saint Christopher, was founded in

1517. In 1524, the first society of noblemen against the custom of toasting was formed in Heidelberg – the Order of the Golden Ring. Luther also criticised the excessive consumption of alcohol in his explanation of Psalm 101 in 1534: "Every country must have its own devil, our German devil must be a big wine drinker called 'Boozer', who is so thirsty that his thirst cannot be quenched with great drinking parties of beer and wine ...."[23] In 1541 he wrote: "Unfortunately the whole of Germany is plagued by drink. We preach ... and complain about it but it doesn't help much ... Emperors, Kings, Rulers and the nobility should do all they could to oppose this."[23]

Despite all these warnings and despite the ideal of moderation, the 16th century was a period of exceptionally high alcohol consumption. It was in this century that brandy lost its purely medicinal application and became extremely popular as a way of becoming intoxicated much more quickly and much more severely than by drinking wine. Moreover, the stronger anaesthetizing effect of brandy had the advantage of thoroughly suppressing any feelings of guilt that might arise (as a result of the immoderate consumption).

Thus, on the one hand, we come across the emergence of the ideals of self-control and moderation in the 16th century while, on the other hand, there was also a conflicting excessive consumption of alcohol, probably as a sort of valve for allowing the inner tensions resulting from self-control to escape.[24] In contrast with the original Dionysus cult, when self-control and the inhibition of feelings were practised during the state of drunkenness, drunkenness now acquired the opposite function: inhibitions were cast off, so that the drinker could let himself go for a while and momentarily abandon the self-control which had been imposed. This still took place on legitimate occasions and with a sense of responsibility for the acts performed while in a drunken state. A Dutch proverb dating from this period goes: "Drunken sins, sober penance".[24]

What were the penalties? In Germany these included: sobering up on bread and water, a three guilder fine, or three days of bread and water for violating the toasting prohibition, being sent to penal institutions or work houses, banishment, the withdrawal of licences for innkeepers and publicans who served alcohol on Sundays, who gave too much credit or who abused alcoholics or drank too much themselves.[25] We do not know whether these punishments were actually imposed but, during the course of the 16th and 17th centuries, there was a gradual decline in the consumption of alcohol partly because other drugs, such as coffee, tea and tobacco began to appear. In 1673, Increase Mathers expressed the puritanical attitude to the consumption of alcohol as follows: "In itself, drink is one of God's good creations and should be gratefully received, but the abuse of drink comes from Satan; wine comes from God but the drunkard from the Devil."[26]

In the following period – up to the Industrial Revolution at the beginning of the 19th century – the trend towards moderation continued even though there were huge waves of excessive alcohol consumption, particularly among the lower classes. One example is the gigantic increase in the consumption of gin in England at the beginning of the 18th century. Some of the figures indicate what happened: the consumption of gin rose from 7.5 million litres in 1714 to more than 40 million litres in 1750. Why was this?

About a century earlier English soldiers had come across the drink, jenever, on their campaigns in the Netherlands. This drink gave them "Dutch courage". When they took it back home, English brewers soon learned to make a similar drink, gin, from grain. At first this was unable to compete with the wine and brandy imported from France but, when William of Orange came to the English throne in 1688 and prohibited the importation of these French products a year later, this paved the way for the introduction of gin. The consumption of this new drug increased slowly from about 2 million litres in 1685 to about 7.5 million litres in 1714; after that it spread rapidly. In 1736 a committee wrote: "People in the lower classes of society drink (gin) uninhibitedly so that at the end of the week they have no money left to take home to their families which starve or fall on the mercy of the council ... With regard to women we have found that the epidemic has even spread amongst them. Unhappy mothers become addicted to it. The children are born weak and sickly and often look emaciated and old as though they are much older than their real age ... the gin drinkers commit many violent crimes and sometimes fall into terrible rages. Children are left at home starved and naked so that they either become a burden on the council ... or are even forced to start begging at a very young age, learning to steal and rob as they get older."[27] Things got really out of hand, particularly in London. Henry Fielding, the famous English playwright, satirist, social reformer, who became a magistrate, wrote in a report in 1751 that: "One of the main causes of poverty and the ensuing criminality is the poison called gin. I have good reasons to assume that it is the main source of sustenance of more than 100,000 people in this city."[27]

After a few failed attempts to pass effective legislation (such as taxing gin in 1729, which merely had the result that good quality gin largely disappeared to be replaced by a much more poisonous inferior sort of brandy, "Parliament brandy"), Parliament decided in 1751, partly as a result of Henry Fielding's report, to introduce some far-reaching measures. For example, distillers were prohibited from trading in alcoholic drinks or selling these on to retailers who did not have a licence. In addition, it became much more difficult to acquire a licence and much stricter penalties were imposed for violations of the law. This reduced supply of gin soon produced results. In the years following 1751 the consumption gradually fell again to 7.5 million litres. By about 1790 the consumption had been reduced to approximately 4 million litres per year. Under the pressure of these measures, many people switched to the new drugs, coffee and tea: by about 1765 it is estimated that nine out of ten families drank tea twice a day.

By the time of the Industrial Revolution (19th century) the general attitude to the use of alcohol was still the same. Aldo Legnaro described this as follows: "... thus, the dominant culture still prescribed that the controlled behaviour in the sense of sober reliability had a functional value in society. Intoxication retained its ambivalent quality which it had acquired at the beginning of the new age (approximately 1500), when it was seen as a forbidden fruit: although it was permitted to 'taste' drink, and it was even necessary to free oneself temporarily from the stringent need to control one's feelings, this could only be done within the narrow limitations of permissible places and times. Anyone who became intoxicated too often, too long and too intensely, would be rejected and was only allowed back into society after publicly expressing remorse and paying the price and promising to be converted."[28] This ambivalence also applied in the Netherlands: "Until the late 19th century ... consumption in festive moderation was considered as a positive and even healthy past-time but alcohol abuse was condemned."[29] In fact, for a few centuries the consumption of alcohol was permitted not only in inns, taverns and other public places but also within the family. Aldo Legnaro wrote: "It is a characteristic feature of the new age that excessive alcohol consumption is becoming a private matter and is therefore permitted within the intimate primary group, above all, the family."[30]

With the Industrial Revolution there were great changes in the working and living conditions of large parts of the population. Many labourers, craftsmen and other people who had become unemployed left the impoverished countryside to seek work in the factories in the growing industrial centres. If they were able to find work the working conditions were atrocious: twelve- to sixteen-hour days, working Sundays, no holidays, dirty air, filthy drinking water, dangerous machinery, extremely low wages. The living conditions were also miserable: one- or two-room dwellings – usually very sparsely furnished – for the entire family, (often sublet to others to earn a little extra).

Therefore it is not surprising that for these people brandy – and to a lesser extent potato gin – were often the only consolation. In 1845, Friedrich Engels wrote: "Every temptation and every enticement combined to encourage the workers to drink. Brandy is virtually the only source of joy for them. Quite apart from the physical conditions which encourage the workers to drink, the knowledge that it is possible to forget the misery and pressures of life for at least a few hours has such a strong effect that one really cannot blame the workers for their predilection for brandy."[31] Many workers started to drink alcoholic drinks so that they would not become ill from the poor quality drinking water, and another significant factor was that workers were often paid part of their wages in the form of brandy, a custom which had started in the alcohol industry and which was adopted by many manufacturers and land owners. Stehr wrote: "This method of paying part of the workers' wages in brandy spread rapidly and soon the transport and building industries, the owners of coal mines and steelworks and of brickworks and tyre factories in Germany also started to do this ..."[31]

An important reason for this was the fact that the technically greatly improved and growing alcohol industry was seeking new customers and found them particularly in the impoverished industrial labouring masses. In addition, there was also an increase in alcohol consumption by soldiers and in the higher and middle classes, while surfeit supplies and inferior products were exported to the native populations of the African colonies.[32]

It was quite a while before it became clear, in the increasingly industrial society with ever more complex technical machinery, that industrial production could not be combined with working under the influence of alcohol. Eventually factory owners realized that "the performance of workers who had a tendency to drink was below the norm."[31]

Therefore, from that time (approximately the middle of the last century) they no longer paid part of the wages in brandy.

Meanwhile, campaigns had been introduced in England, Scotland, Ireland, Sweden and America to oppose the abuse of spirits. In 1842 the Dutch Association for the Abolition of Liquor was founded in the Netherlands. As its name suggests, this body was opposed only to the consumption of strong liquor, i.e. the use of distilled alcohol such as brandy and gin. It did not cover beer and wine because the risks entailed by these were not yet recognized. In fact, ale houses were even established to reduce the consumption of distilled alcohol. The Dutch Association had a growing number of members: from 1,834 members in 1843 (a year after its establishment) to 14,000 in 1867. However, despite all its efforts, the consumption of spirits continued to rise. They were swimming against the tide and, in 1854, the Association's annual report concluded: "The lower classes drink and continue to drink whatever they are told, however convinced they are of the misery which they inflict upon themselves."[33] The consumption of alcohol continued to rise up to the 1870s, but then the tide turned. In 1881 the first teetotal association was founded. The members voiced their objections not only to distilled spirits, but also to the production, trade and consumption of all other alcoholic drinks (including beer and wine). In 1894 teetotallers could also become members of the Dutch Association for the Abolition of Liquor, and by 1899 the principle of the abolition of spirits was changed by the Association into a principle of complete abstinence. This encountered some objections but "the insight grew that beer, wine and so on also led to drunkenness and dangers, and were possibly just as harmful. There was also the feeling that it was not right to continue drinking oneself while the lower classes had to do without."[33]

In addition, a strong feeling against the abuse of alcohol by the working classes developed in the rising socialist movement. Wherever workers organized themselves and acquired power there was a reduction in the consumption of alcohol. Domela Nieuwenhuis spoke his famous words: "Drinking workers do not think and thinking workers do not drink", and this certainly produced some results.

As a result there was a strong movement against alcohol which came from different levels of society. It was a real movement of the people which enthusiastically opposed "the demon drink, Satan's beverage, the plague of gin or the monster of alcohol", and either wanted to prohibit it altogether, or aimed to prohibit some alcohol (spirits) or tried to urge people to drink in moderation. The movement was successful. The first Drinking Act was passed in 1881, restricting the sale of spirits to a limited number of licences which helped to achieve a slow decline in the total consumption of alcohol (except distilled drink). The decline rapidly gained momentum after 1900 (even in distilled drinks). This decline continued up to the end of the Second World War (see graph 1 on page 26). An important element in this process, apart from changing attitudes, was the second Drinking Act of 1904 which provided that even the vendors of weak alcoholic drinks (beer and wine), henceforth required a licence from the local council, and that young people under the age of sixteen could not enter a cafe or off-licence unless they were accompanied by someone who was over twenty-one. By 1917 the movement had grown to such an extent that there were an estimated sixty-thousand teetotallers, sixty-thousand "abolitionists" (who only prohibited distilled drink), and twenty-seven-thousand moderates who were actively involved. However, in the following years the social interest in opposing drink gradually cooled in the Netherlands because of the success that had been achieved.

It was entirely different in another country, viz. Finland, the first European country to completely prohibit the consumption of alcohol (in 1919). From 1919 to 1930 the consumption of alcohol doubled there. The number of men who were arrested every year in Helsinki for public drunkenness rose to one third (25,000) of the adult male population. Alcohol was involved in 40% of all accidents – a quarter of these were stabbings, and the percentage of patients admitted to psychiatric institutions with alcohol problems rose from 8% in 1919 to 28% in 1931. In 1931 the Act was withdrawn.

A much more successful approach to counteracting the consumption of alcohol was the introduction of drastic price increases (taxation on alcohol), which took place in Sweden and Denmark. In Sweden the consumption fell by 50% as a result and in Denmark by a quarter. In that country the number of chronic alcoholics/patients suffering from delirium tremens fell from 40 per 100,000 inhabitants in 1910 to 2 per 100,000 inhabitants in 1935.

After the Second World War there was an increase in the consumption of alcohol. This increase mushroomed spectacularly during the

1960s. In the second half of the 1970s it levelled off and for a short while there was even a slight reduction (see the graphs and explanation in chapter 3).[34]

Before concluding this account of how alcohol is currently related to the social and economic structures of a number of European countries, we would first like to focus our attention on the country which was first overpowered by alcohol and which then tried to overpower alcohol itself by means of prohibition, i.e. America.

The white colonists in the 16th century introduced alcohol to America. The native Americans were not familiar with this drink, though they appreciated the taste, and proved to be extremely susceptible to it: they reacted much more strongly than the white colonists to the same quantities of alcohol. They called alcohol "wisakon" (it is bitter) or "eskotewapo" (fire water). Their word for the rum which was often used became "milk" or "mother's milk". During the first few hundred years alcohol was used mainly for bartering for furs. For example, in 1770 the white traders bartered four fifths of all furs from the Chickasaws for rum.

However, the native Americans were not able to resist the effects of alcohol. In 1698 Delaware spoke to white colonists in New Jersey: "We know that it is harmful for us to drink. We know it but when you sell us alcohol, it controls us to such an extent that we are unable to refuse it. When we drink alcohol it turns us into savages; we don't know what we are doing, we injure each other, we throw each other into the fire. Seven of our tribes have died out as a result of drinking brandy."[35]

In order to restrict these consequences of drunkenness and the consequent aggression as much as possible, many native American tribes took measures. For example, they provided every drinker with one or two members of the tribe to monitor them and to prevent the drinker from becoming aggressive and destructive. Sometimes a group of warriors was detailed to keep order and after collecting everyone's weapons they banished every drinker who misbehaved from the group. However, these measures did not help much. The Frenchman Bougainville wrote in 1758: "A drunken man is a holy man"[36] and this reflected the general view which prevailed amongst many native American tribes. He described the goal of their drinking as complete intoxication rather than the acquisition of a degree of freedom: "They saturated themselves with brandy, drank litres at a time and let go of the bottle only when they fell to the ground in a stupor. In their eyes there is no more beautiful death than death from alcohol poisoning. Drinking is their paradise."[36]

As stated above, the native Americans did not have any tolerance against alcohol, which was a foreign substance for their bodies and their culture. In fact, they were also unable to drink milk (apart from mother's milk), a drink which they did not know and could not tolerate. They did not consider themselves responsible for the consequences of their consumption, but considered the alcohol to be responsible. It was not the drinker, but the alcohol which was guilty of their aggressive and criminal actions. It was not they, but the white traders, who should pay the price for the consequences of consumption. Official attempts were occasionally taken to drastically reduce or even prohibit the trade in alcohol. This finally "succeeded" in 1832, but it was to little avail because there was always a trader somewhere who would provide the desired liquor in return for furs. Christian F. Feest wrote: "In their colony, Alaska, the Russians strictly prohibited the trade in brandy but smugglers from New England soon took over. When the French stopped supplying drink in the region of the Great Lakes, the British replaced them with barrels of rum. When the British stopped they had to take into account the fact that the French would acquire significant advantages in the fur trade as a result of gifts of alcohol."[37]

Alcohol gradually tore the native Americans away from their links with the supernatural world. Alcohol destroyed the connection with the divine and spiritual world in their consciousness. Because they lost this relationship with the world of the gods, the social structures gradually broke down – at least in those tribes who used alcohol (and continued to use it). The ancient relations between tribes dissolved and the native Americans were left isolated from each other. Many were unable to tolerate the consequent psychological and social disintegration – combined with the diseases and psychological breakdown caused by alcohol – and committed suicide. In addition, many died as a result of the diseases caused by alcohol consumption or as a result of the bloody conflicts and tribal warfare encouraged by alcohol. Schmidbauer and Vom Scheidt wrote that the population of North American Indians was decimated by the use of alcohol.[38]

In 17th and 18th century America, white colonists drank a lot of alocohol (especially rum).[39] It was taken in small quantities with meals, during lunch, before going to sleep, and so on, but also in large quantities at communal celebrations such as harvest festivals, parties, births, birthdays etc. although they did not see this as a problem. For most Americans "intoxication" was a natural and innocent consequence of drinking.[40] It was felt that many people got drunk because they wanted to and not because they had to. Alcohol was not seen as affecting the will or leading to addiction. In other words, people drank because they liked drinking and not because they were unable to do without.

This changed by the end of the 18th and the beginning of the 19th century. There were some Americans who admitted that they felt an overpowering and irresistible desire for alcohol, and that they were no longer in control of themselves in this respect. For example, in 1795, there was a man who made a declaration under oath begging everyone not to sell him alcohol because "this bad habit had seriously impaired his faculties and injured his person and it was not possible for him to give up this habit unless if it was impossible to obtain alcohol."[41] Many such declarations were made. Instead of referring to a "liking" or "predilection" for alcohol it was described in terms of an "overwhelming", "irresistible", "destructive" desire for alcohol. The concept of alcohol addiction was introduced at about the same time as it was in Europe. Benjamin Rush was the first person to interpret this concept in a modern way. He described alcohol addiction as a disease, a disease of the will: "The habit of drinking too much is initially a decision of the free will. From a habit it becomes a necessity."[42] He illustrated this inability to refrain from drinking, this loss of self-control, as follows: "When a habitual drinker was implored by one of his friends to stop drinking he said: 'If there were a barrel of rum in the corner of the room and if a cannon constantly fired cannonballs between me and the barrel, I still could not stop myself from walking past the cannon to get to the barrel of rum!'"[42]

According to Rush, the only remedy was complete abstinence: "On the basis of my observations I can say that alcoholics must stop drinking completely and immediately. In the house of a man who wishes to be cured of drinking, every bottle which contains alcohol should be labelled 'Don't try it, don't pick it up, don't touch it'"[42] With these words Rush became the theoretical founder of the radical Temperance Movement in the United States, a movement which advocated complete abstinence and which, after a slow start at the beginning of the 19th century, grew to become a massive popular movement with half a million members in 1835 and many millions of members later on.[43] In this movement the notion prevailed that it was alcohol and not the drinker which was the cause of all evil. As for the native Americans alcohol was blamed for all disease, poverty, aggression, criminality, insanity and broken homes.

This formed the basis for prohibition, which will be described in detail below, but for the time being a great deal of attention was devoted to the victims of alcohol as well as the propaganda for complete abstinence. There was an attempt to empathise with the drinker and to help him in his struggle against the demon alcohol. One member of the Temperance Movement wrote (1833): "We have all seen such cases in which a longer or shorter period of complete abstinence is followed by an attack of deadly weakness... when they are sober, they can honestly assess their own situation and the danger they are in: they know that it is not possible for them to drink moderately. They decide to abstain communally and in that way avoid the temptation because they are too weak to resist it. Slowly they gain self-confidence and feel secure in their own ability to resist. Then they try a sip of wine. From that moment the balance of self-control which has just been achieved is once again disrupted, the demon returns, common sense is driven out and the person is ruined."[43]

Therefore the only remedy seemed to be complete and permanent abstinence. The arguments for this were formulated in 1830 and continued to apply throughout the whole of the 19th century and part of the 20th century. These arguments were:

"1. Alcohol is an addictive substance. Although it is initially harmless, the desire to drink increases until a state of complete dependence is reached. Habitual drinking and alcohol addiction are the normal consequences of the regular consumption of alcohol.

2. The direct affect of alcohol consists of weakening the drinker's moral consciousness and self-control. Alcohol gives rise to animal passions and acts of violence. A significant proportion of poverty and criminality (about three-quarters) must be attributed to the moral degeneration resulting from the use of alcohol.

3. Alcohol is a poison and weakens both the complete physical constitution and the mental and moral faculties. Alcohol is the direct cause of many diseases and renders the body susceptible to many other diseases."[44]

To summarize and review these points, Harry Gene Levine formulates the view generally held in the Temperance Movement as follows: "Poverty, criminality, slums, abandoned women and children, business failures and personal downfall were not the result of wrongful developments in the economy and in society, according to the beliefs of the Temperance Movement, but were the results of alcohol. Alcohol was the scapegoat in the classical sense of the word: a victim which had to be judged to liberate society from its greatest suffering and problems. America would be healthy if the nation completely abstained."[45] (cf. the war on drugs in our own time.)

Initially it was attempted to achieve this goal by means of education and by encouraging everyone to stop drinking or not to start in the first place. However, by about 1850, many people within the movement had come to the conclusion that their goal could only be achieved by placing a complete prohibition on alcoholic drinks.

Some attempts were made to change the legislation accordingly (in about 1850 and 1880) but these did not lead to the desired permanent results. The campaign became even more intense and professional in the 20th century. The Anti-Saloon-League, which had grown from the Temperance Movement, made use of the most modern methods of political pressure and lobbying. Many professionals in this organization addressed politicians, submitted draft laws and actively advised people to vote for politicians who clearly supported the complete prohibition of alcohol during their election campaigns, almost always with decisive effect. This strategy worked very well: in the first decade of the 20th century many cities, councils and states gradually became "dry".

The next step followed in 1913: the campaign for a national prohibition on alcohol. The targets were in the first place the powerful distilling industry and the bars, particularly in cities, which were seen not only as centres of drinking, but also as hotbeds where subversive and communist plots were hatched by dissident workers and immigrants (hence the name "Anti-Saloon-League"). Influential industrialists such as John D. Rockefeller joined this campaign; sober workers would work harder, operate the machines better, take less sick leave and have fewer industrial accidents, demand lower wages and strike less (because they no longer needed money for their alcohol consumption). Moreover, the workers would be able to spend their money on consumer articles which would benefit the economy as a whole. Taxes could come down because less money would have to be spent on the police, prisons, courts, hospitals and so on which were all needed as a result of the criminality, poverty, corruption, disease and accidents caused by drinking.

By the early 1920s the goal was achieved and America was dry.

The Anti-Saloon-League declared: "A new nation will be born". Certainly the consumption of alcohol declined in this new nation, at least amongst workers, but it was also a nation of illegal moonshiners, bootleggers and rum runners, illegal saloons, night clubs, gangster mobs, corrupt police and politicians. The alcohol was of an inferior quality and sometimes lethal: in 1930 it is estimated that there were approximately 15,000 people whose legs had been paralysed as a result of drinking a very poisonous strong alcoholic drink – so called Jake Jazz. Above all, there was a spectacular rise in criminality. Contempt for the law was in danger of becoming the norm. Furthermore, America gained a bad name abroad.

It was because of these developments that a group of authoritative, wealthy and very influential people – almost all of them major industrialists – formed the AAPA, the Association Against the Prohibition Amendment in 1926. This was aimed at ending prohibition. The board of directors of this group included many directors and managing directors of large companies such as American Telephone and Telegraph, Southern Pacific Railroad, Goodrich Rubber, Anaconda Copper, US Steel, General Electric, Phillips and Boeing. They were led by Pierre Du Pont (Dupont Chemicals) and John J. Raskob (General Motors). This was "a group which had more money behind it than all the propaganda campaigns ever held in the world all together".[46]

Why did they do this? In his article "The Temperance Movement and prohibition in the USA",[46] Harry Gene Levine listed the three following reasons:

1. They believed that a reintroduction of taxation on alcoholic drinks would lead to a general reduction in taxation which would be to their advantage as well as to that of their companies. The increased taxation which had accompanied prohibition (because the treasury no longer had any income from the alcohol industry) would therefore be reversed.

2. They believed that the lawlessness and deterioration of norms resulting from prohibition would eventually lead to a general loss of respect for the law and to the end of law-abiding behaviour which was extremely dangerous for public order.

3. They believed that the reintroduction of the alcohol industry would result in many hundreds of thousands of jobs and an income for municipalities and states which would be a welcome development particularly during those years of economic recession and extremely high unemployment.

In 1932, the lowest point of the economic crisis, John D. Rockefeller changed from being a supporter to an opponent of prohibition because of his fear of the collapse of the law. In the same year the democrats led by Franklin D. Roosevelt who had made the abolition of prohibition one of the major policies of his election campaign, won the election and the deed was soon done. On 16 February 1933 the Prohibition Act (the Prohibition Amendment) was revoked by the Senate (63 votes against 23) and four days later by the House of Representatives (289 against 121). The "newborn" nation had lasted all of fourteen years and had lost many illusions. The prisons were overcrowded and there were applications for hundreds of new prisons. The justice system was completely over-burdened (there were applications for thousands of additional officers of justice because they could no longer cope with the work), the underworld had gained an enormous amount of power and tens of thousands of deaths resulted from the consumption of lethal alcoholic substances. All in all the belief in the possibility of recreating society had disappeared and a more realistic approach was adopted.

Following the repeal of prohibition, the production of alcoholic drinks was soon taken over by a few huge concerns. As a result the quality of the alcohol improved and the number of alcohol-related deaths fell in New York from 794 in 1931 to 509 in 1935. The alcohol industry expanded rapidly and within three years it had returned to the former level although the people in America itself drank less (60% of the consumption before prohibition), a trend which paralleled that in Holland. By 1940 there were more than a million people working in the alcohol industry, trade and sales; the consumption of alcohol was fully re-integrated into American society and has not been a matter of political importance since that time.

To conclude this description of the history of alcohol with an idea of how alcohol has been integrated into western society, it is appropriate to examine the two largest wine-producing countries in the world, viz. France and Italy.

In France:
- viniculture is responsible for 11% of all the agricultural income,
- the revenue from wine amounts to 17 billion French francs per year.

In Italy:
- two million people are wholly or partly dependant on the production or sale of wine for their income,

– approximately 10% of agricultural land is used for viniculture.

However, the other side of the coin is that 20,000-30,000 people die in France every year as a result of cirrhosis of the liver, delirium tremens and degeneration of the kidneys.

Looking back, we see how mankind has struggled for centuries with the gift from Dionysus, a struggle which continues today and which has merely increased in size and intensity since the protective strength of tradition has collapsed. Now that alcohol addiction – and the collapse of tradition – is a fact, we see how every person in the western world is individually exposed to the alcohol phenomenon. Alcohol has gained a much greater influence on people and can make its effects felt much more powerfully. Prohibitions no longer help, except extremely strict prohibitions, such as those in the orthodox Muslim countries. Therefore, everyone has to establish their own relationship with what is the most common hard drug in the world on the basis of his own individual consciousness (at least in countries where these prohibitions do not apply).

An insight into the effects of alcohol can be helpful in this respect. That is why we will try to describe the effect of alcohol on human beings as clearly as possible below. Before we do this, we will start by examining what alcohol actually is and how it is made.

How is alcohol produced?

Alcohol is the result of fermentation. What does this mean and how does this work? In order to describe it, we must look at the preparation of wine because the process of fermentation for producing the oldest alcoholic drink of all takes place under particularly favourable conditions.

As soon as the grapes on the vine are sufficiently ripe they are picked, crushed and – after removing the pips and stalks – they are placed in tubs where the natural fermentation process of the grape juice starts. While the fruit was forming, numerous spores settled on the skins of the grapes, and these now start to multiply uninhibitedly in the sweet grape juice. As a result, the grape juice undergoes the "turbulent" process of fermentation and the grape sugar is converted into alcohol, while carbon dioxide is released. Red wine is made from black grapes which have fermented with their skins for 10 to 15 days; rosé is made from black grapes when the skins are fermented with the grape juice for 12 to 24 hours; white wine is made by allowing the grapes to ferment without their skins. The fermentation comes

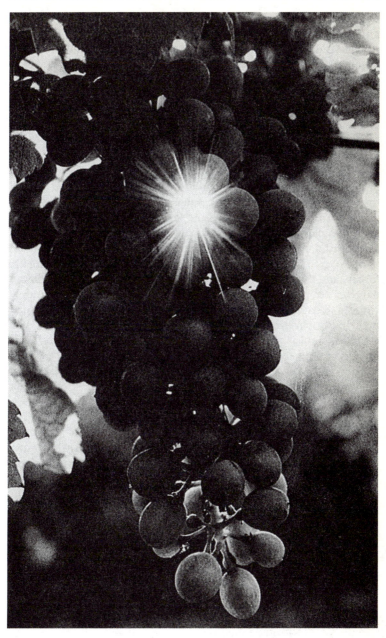

Photograph: Grapes, one of the raw materials for alcohol.

to an end when the alcohol which has been produced destroys the fermenting agents which cannot live where the percentage of alcohol is higher than 10-15 per cent. In this way alcohol destroys the vegetable elements to which it owes its existence. Lower plant life forms (fermenting agents) destroy higher plant life forms (the grape) and in this destruction the fermented cells also destroy themselves. What remains from this process of destruction and death, apart from a few waste products, is alcohol. This is permanent.[47]

Looking at this process in another light reveals the following fact. The vine has assimilated many vital forces (life forces) in the grapes in the course of its development as it ripens in the light and heat of the sun. The grapes – and their sugars and vitamins – are therefore very nutritious and have a vitalising regenerative effect on us and are good for cleaning the blood. They strengthen our life forces by transferring some of the vitality and growing power contained in them to us. The fruit is permeated with forces of growth, strong life forces, and the primitive lower plant life of the fermenting cells can develop tempestuously in these forces of growth. They multiply without restraint and destroy the fruit by means of the one-sided breaking down process of metabolism – as do mushrooms.[48] As a result, alcohol is produced, mummifying the grape juice and conserving and preserving it in the form of wine.[49]

Under less favourable circumstances (i.e. with some other fruit containing sugar and brewing grains) the above-mentioned process of fermentation has been used in the history of western culture to produce other alcoholic drinks. In the first place there is beer which is obtained by fermenting the malt[50] of barley, together with water, brewer's yeast and hops. Beer owes its taste partly to the hop plant.
    Since the early Middle Ages there has also been a distillation technique for producing drinks with a higher alcohol percentage, as was described in the history of alcohol. These drinks include:
- brandy, obtained by distilling wine;
- cognac, distilled from wine and kept for a long time in oak barrels;
- reinforced wines, such as port, where alcohol has been added;
- gin and jenever, distilled from grains over juniper berries until the specific taste is achieved;
- whisky, distilled from a fermented mixture of rye and barley malt, obtaining the aroma by storing it for a long time in wooden barrels with a carbonized lining;

- rum, obtained by distilling sugar cane molasses;
- vodka, distilled from potatoes.

All these drinks have their specific qualities, so that the consumer nowadays can choose which alcoholic drug will suit him best at a particular time in his life depending on his personal circumstances, needs and preferences. However, what they all have in common, despite the differences in quality, is alcohol.

The effects of alcohol

First, it must be noted that there is always a small amount of alcohol present in the human body. The human body produces this alcohol itself in the liver.[51] There is also a small amount of alcohol in the blood. This minimal quantity of alcohol amounts to approximately 0.001 parts per thousand.[52]

What happens when a person imbibes alcohol? The alcohol enters the blood directly and to a greater or lesser extent, depending on the amount consumed, reaches all the organs of the human body through the mucus membrane in the mouth and the stomach and intestinal walls.

In the blood the additional quantity of alcohol acts as a sort of tap or "bomb"; the natural level of parts per 1000 is overwhelmed and after 1 or 2 glasses of alcohol it rises to 0.1–0.4 parts per 1000, after 3 to 4 glasses to 0.5–0.6 parts per thousand, and after 5 to 6 glasses to 0.7–1.0 parts per thousand. After 9 to 10 glasses it rises to 1.7–2.0 parts per thousand, and after to 11–15 glasses to 2.1–3.9 parts per thousand. More than 26 glasses (more than 5.1 parts per thousand) results in death through heart failure.[53]

When alcohol is assimilated, after a few glasses the circulation of the blood accelerates, the heartbeat speeds up and blood pressure rises. It is as though the alcohol causes the same turbulent processes in the blood as those to which it owes its existence.

Many people experience this foaming "fermenting effect" of a few glasses of alcohol as a (slight) excitement. In the first instance, alcohol has a stimulating effect; it also increases the rate of respiration as well as its depth. The rhythmic system is activated and the astral body is more closely linked to the digestive organs (particularly the kidneys, which is why the blood pressure increases) and the circulation.

The drinker starts moving and gets going. His emotions are released and everything starts to flow. This is the reason why writers such as Faulkner and Hemingway drank alcohol before they started work.

However, at the same time, the astral body withdraws. Alcohol has an inhibitory effect on the central and peripheral nervous systems and paralyses the nerves of the peripheral arteries. This has the result that the blood vessels of the skin and muscles become weaker and wider which leads to bleeding under the skin (red eyes, nose and face). This paralysing effect of alcohol on the nervous system warms the drinker; for example, after a strong drink or a good glass of cognac he feels comfortably warm even if it is quite cold. He no longer feels the cold of the outside world, because the sensitivity to heat has been cancelled out. As the peripheral blood vessels no longer contract under the influence of the cold, this can result in a life-threatening situation in extremely cold conditions, as too much body heat is lost through the blood-gorged skin. The drinker cools off rapidly without noticing it. Many people who have gone outside to sleep off their drunkenness in the cold have died because their body temperature fell below the critical level.

Thus we see that alcohol has an extremely strong effect on the circulation and on the body heating system. What does this mean when we examine the effects of alcohol in more detail in relation to the essential aspects of humankind?

In the first place the body heating system is the physical basis for the Self. In *Antroposofische geneeskunde* (Anthroposophical Medicine), Victor Bott wrote: "The spirit (the Self) has a physical base, as do the other bodies – this is the heating system. If it were possible to isolate the heat of our body, we would see that this is not the same everywhere but that it has a structure and an organization (an organization which can actually be partly revealed in infra-red photographs). Therefore, it is perfectly justified to refer to the 'heating organism' which allows the Self to function".[54] He expresses this in the following series: Self (or human spirit); organic support: heating organism; natural element: fire.[54]

As regards the ethereal body, the Self also has a supporting function in the principle of heat. Bernard Lievegoed wrote: "The effect of ethereal heat permeates the total organism. It has its central organ in the circulation of the blood and it is the medium through which man's spiritual Self can come into contact with the living, physical body".[55]

Therefore, man's Self can manifest itself on earth – through ethereal heat – in the heating organism, in which the warm circulation of the blood, with the heart as the central organ, is the most important medium. This blood, this instrument of the Self, is changed through the effect of alcohol; its rhythm is disrupted.

Rudolf Steiner wrote: "Which essential aspect of man is influenced when he drinks alcohol? It is the Self, of which the physical instruments are the blood and the circulation. The circulation of the blood in man which gives him life is greatly influenced by alcohol".[56]

The heating organism is also partly paralysed, as stated above, and loses its equilibrium. The warmth flows out into the outside world with the result that the true – spiritual – Self can no longer manifest itself optimally in man's disrupted heating and circulation organism; the manifestation of the Self to the world is affected.

In the case of repeated use, this can obviously result in a situation where the impulses and development of the Self find it more difficult to manifest themselves, or are manifest in a distorted or reduced fashion. In this case, the person's development is in danger of stagnating. Increasingly he starts to repeat himself, remains unchanged and preserves the status quo.

A closer look at the process of the influence on the instrument of the Self – on the blood – by the use of alcohol also shows a change in the blood sugar level resulting from the use of alcohol.

During the process of digestion the human organism produces its own sugar in the liver, from, inter alia, drinks containing sugar (such as grape juice and fruit juices) and from foods rich in carbohydrates (such as bread and cereals). This circulates round the body in the form of blood sugar and is present everywhere, including the brain and muscular tissues, i.e. it penetrates the whole body. When the body is saturated with this sugar, any extra sugar serves for the creation of glycogen, a starchy substance which is stored in the liver or in the cells of the muscles and which can in turn be converted into sugar when necessary. In addition, the human organism produces glucose (sugar) in the liver from amino acids amongst other things: this process is known as glyconeogenesis.

In this way the human organism produces the required amount of blood sugar. In a healthy person this is always at a constant level. A strong reduction in the blood sugar level leads to shock and life threatening situations resulting in unconsciousness.[57]

An examination of the blood sugar content in relation to the essential aspects of human beings reveals that blood sugar is just as important as blood heat because "the highest aspect of man, the Self, the spiritual core, needs this sugar as a tool to develop his impulses in the body."[58]

"The blood sugar is the carrier of the Self."[57] In this context, Rudolf Steiner and Ita Wegman wrote: "While the blood, containing sugar, circulates through the whole body, it carries the organization of the Self through the body." They also wrote: "Where there is sugar, there is an organization of the Self ..."[59] (The organization of the Self refers to the organization which the Self has imposed on the essential aspects over the course of time and in which the Self can reveal itself and manifest itself. The Self manifests itself in the organization of the Self.)

The blood sugar level is often changed by the effect of alcohol. Following the breakdown of alcohol (oxidation) in the liver, first of all there is an inhibiting effect on the process of glyconeogenesis or the potential formation of new sugar.[60] This can result in hypoglycaemia (a reduced blood sugar level), which is one of the most common complications in cases of acute alcohol poisoning.[61] When there are no other possibilities of producing blood sugar, which is often the case in alcoholics,[62] the inhibition of glyconeogenesis can lead to serious problems (including fits).

However, the opposite can also happen; the effect of alcohol can temporarily reduce the symptoms of hypoglycaemia (tremors),[63] while there may also be an increase in the blood sugar level particularly in the case of long-term consumption, as a result of a combination of other factors.[64]

In short, the effect of alcohol can lead to a change in the normal blood sugar level; an increase in the blood sugar level (as in diabetes) is generally less dangerous than a decrease in the level.

However, an increase in the blood sugar level is also unfavourable because when this happens the Self has a much less efficient tool for developing its impulses in the body.

The change in the blood sugar level brought about by alcohol and the related partial obstruction or breakdown of the organization of the Self, in addition to the effects on the systems responsible for body heat and circulation, can have a number of far-reaching effects on the consumer:

a. In the first place, the partial breakdown of the organization of the Self leads to the expulsion of the Self's life forces. They rise up, so that the consumer feels as though he is (slightly) raised above the earthly plane; he feels looser, lighter and freer.

b. However, as a result, the Self is less able to gain access to the person who is under the influence of alcohol. It temporarily shuts itself off, to a greater or lesser extent, from its spiritual origins and its essential spiritual core. In a spiritual sense, it becomes more or less isolated and alienated from the essential being.

c. There is another aspect. Rudolf Steiner and Ita Wegman wrote: "Where there is sugar, there is an organization of the Self; when sugar is produced, the organization of the Self acts to give a direction to the subhuman (vegetative, animal) aspect of the body towards the human aspect."[59] This quote can be slightly changed: where there is sugar, there is an organization of the Self; when there is an inhibiting effect on the production of (blood) sugar, the organization of the Self cannot act as effectively in directing the subhuman (vegetative = ethereally determined), animal (= astrally determined) body towards the human aspect.

This reduced effectiveness of the organization of the Self is easy to see in the inhibiting effect which alcohol has on the process of glyconeogenesis. As soon as the liver starts to break down the alcohol and produces the first poisonous waste product (acetaldehyde) glyconeogenesis is immediately inhibited, i.e. there is an inhibition of the new blood sugar from amino acids amongst other things.

Thus the organization of the Self is less effective as a result of alcohol. This has a number of consequences:

– The animal emotional forces of the consumer's astral body have a stronger effect. The drives, desires and passions which are normally controlled in daily life by the organization of the Self become less inhibited: alcohol has an uninhibiting effect. In addition, the metabolic processes taking place in the blood are now less controlled by the organization of the Self and are therefore uninhibited, giving additional force to the drives, emotions and passions. In this case the consumer feels very powerful and may, for example, lose his shyness as a result of the power of the drink. He can feel like a radiant focus, a "sun", and become excessively generous, reckless, or lose self-control. He may want to perform great sexual feats and feel capable of doing anything, while completely over-estimating himself. His astral forces break through forcefully and out of control, individual human qualities recede, sentiments increase (loudly), borders are crossed. Just think of carnival!

– The vegetative physical aspect, i.e. in this case the uncontrolled inhuman forces of the ethereal body, become predominant. This means that the forces resulting from continuously repeating one-self (the ethereal body lives in rhythmic repetitive processes; for example, the consumer may retell the same story over and over again while he is under the influence), of dozing off, of sinking into a passive sentimental consciousness, of becoming apathetic and lazy, all start to predominate, particularly in the case of acute intoxication.

In addition, the patterns of habits, deeper characteristics and personal idiosyncrasies (hobby horses) established in the ethereal body, are now given free rein. Anyone who regularly consumes alcohol develops his own style of intoxication. Van Epen wrote: "In cases of greater poisoning, everyone develops an individual style of intoxication." For example, there is the "sad" and the "aggressive" drunk. One becomes loud and maniacal; the other becomes extremely pathetic.

In every case we see that certain personality traits which are always present – though they are wholly or partly suppressed when a person is sober – become clear and exaggerated under the influence of alcohol. People with a love of ostentation and vanity may irresponsibly give away large sums of money to complete strangers when they are drunk. Others are overcome by feelings of sympathy and empathy and would like to carry the weight of the suffering of the whole world on their shoulders. A typical habit of many people when they are under the influence of large amounts of alcohol is that they often repeat the same story a number of times, using the same words ...."[65]

Thus, the ethereal forces have a stronger influence on the drinker's behaviour. In relation to cognac, Rudolf Steiner wrote: "When a person drinks cognac, his ethereal body has a very strong effect; in fact, this applies to all spirits. He feels comfortable because he switches off his consciousness and becomes rather plant-like. When he has a drink he descends into a vegetative state, and this is a pleasant feeling, just as being asleep is a pleasant feeling, although he is not conscious of this feeling of well-being when he is asleep."[66]

Thus, a person is taking a step backwards when he consumes alcohol. Everything which he has built up during his development with regard to the inter-penetration, individualization and humanization of his astral, ethereal and physical bodies, is temporarily out of action to a greater or lesser extent: he makes an about turn and actually becomes more childlike. He takes the opposite direction of the normal development from childhood to adulthood as, because of the change in the blood sugar level, the organization of the Self is decreasingly able to engage in the humanizing process, i.e. the inner penetration and individualization of the astral, ethereal and physical bodies.

Therefore, the user gradually loses the skills which he has acquired since his earliest youth with the organization of the Self. These are skills such as walking straight, talking, thinking and remembering, skills which are mastered in roughly the first three years of life as typical human qualities – in contrast with animal qualities: walking in the first year of life, talking in the second year, thinking and memory in the third year.

These skills, these qualities of the organization of the Self, are influenced by the consumption of alcohol.

– Thinking becomes sloppier, the thought processes are quicker and associations follow each other at a greater rate, while the critical faculties and the ability to distinguish deteriorate. Large quantities of alcohol result in a virtual disappearance of logic and co-ordination of ideas and the thought processes become increasingly confused. Finally, at a later stage of intoxication, or in cases of very large quantities of alcohol, the ability to think disappears (almost) entirely, consciousness becomes disturbed in the sense of blunted thought processes, stupidity, sleepiness and finally unconsciousness.

– However, before things go this far, the causes of subsequent blackouts have already been laid. Van Epen wrote: "After strong intoxication it is typical for the consumer to have a very faint memory of what exactly happened while he was intoxicated. This phenomenon is known as a blackout."[67] This indicates that during the state of intoxication the Self was no longer (entirely) present; it had departed to a greater or lesser extent, and later on can therefore no longer remember exactly what happened during the state of intoxication. In short, the Self is no longer able to carry out one of its most important functions – memory.[68]

– Speech is affected: initially alcohol loosens the tongue, but even "in a state of light intoxication", words can be used incorrectly and mistakes are made. In addition, heavy intoxication leads to slurred speech.[67] Finally, the consumer can no longer utter a word if he has drunk a huge amount of alcohol – he becomes quite speechless.

– The ability to walk straight and in an upright position decreases as a person becomes more intoxicated; the consumer starts to stagger, stumble, fall over and finally becomes completely unable to stand on his own two legs. It is as though he has become a baby once again and must be carried or transported by car.

This loss of the qualities of the organization of the Self, as well as the reduction or loss of sensory functions such as sight (double vision), hearing, smell, taste, touch, balance, movement (motor co-ordination) and feelings of heat and cold, are also caused by the increasing penetration of alcohol into the brain tissue. In addition, the skills described above and the centres in the brain related to the sensory functions are suppressed, extinguished and consequently switched off to a greater extent. Once again the Self is expelled. The Self – as well as the astral body – can no longer adequately connect with the brain as a result of these disruptions of the brain processes.

Examining the effect of alcohol on the user's astral body it is clear the forces of the Self are no longer able to penetrate the astral body "from above" to the same extent, because of the partial absence of the organization of the Self. On the other hand, the forces of the ethereal and physical body which come from "below" have a much greater influence on the astral body. The astral body is more strongly linked to these and this is a great difference from the effects of opium and hashish, for example. Rudolf Steiner wrote: "When opium is used, the astral body is free from the physical body and thus the user perceives many things, albeit unclearly. He does not have ordinary dreams, but observes the spiritual world. He goes on long journeys through the spiritual world ... People in the east attribute many things which they pass on from the spiritual world, albeit incorrectly, to the use of opium, hashish, etc. In contrast, drinking alcohol takes possession of the physical body, even the blood. This means the astral body cannot be free but is taken over much more by the physical body. That is why man is completely overwhelmed in a physical sense when he drinks alcohol, much more so than in the normal state".[56]

Thus there are various tendencies for the astral body; on the one hand, it is controlled to a much greater extent by the astral forces of pleasure, displeasure, sympathy, antipathy, drives, passions and desires and so on which are present in the astral body, as a result of the partial absence of the organization of the Self, while on the other hand, the forces of metabolism, temperament (ethereal body) and material weight (physical body), which are present in the physical and ethereal bodies, have a much greater influence on the astral body. It is these last two influences from "below" which cause the consumer to become heavier (heavy drunkenness), so that he keeps repeating himself and stagnates.

The use of alcohol by the young

Thus one of the most important effects of alcohol is that it stimulates the astral forces in their crudest form, and that it links these astral forces to the physical body. In this sense it greatly awakens the part of the astral body that has not been "humanized". This is a particular problem for children when they use alcohol. After all, a child's astral body only becomes independent, or is born as it were, at puberty.[69]

If a child drinks alcohol before puberty, its "embryonic" astral body containing latent astral forces is prematurely awakened. The astral forces are stimulated from outside by the alcohol; in fact, the astral body is forced into premature "birth" by the influence of alcohol.

Rudolf Steiner said: "That is why when a child drinks alcohol when it is too young, it acquires an astral body which should only be developing fully at the age of fifteen or sixteen; the child does not have any power over it".[70] It is easy to imagine this because an astral body which is "born" prematurely is like a plaything containing the feelings of pleasure, unhappiness, sympathy, antipathy and so on which have been evoked. It is thrown about, and the very young user cannot control this. He is not yet able to control these feelings and is dragged along by them, which can result in a handicap in later life which is difficult to overcome. As an adult he realizes that he can hardly control his own desires, sympathies, antipathies, wishes, etc. or cannot control them at all, and has a tendency to constantly run after them.

If alcohol is first used during puberty, in other words after the "birth" of the astral body, it will still be a considerable task for a youthful user to learn to control the astral forces which have been unleashed. In fact, this is probably the reason why adolescents drink so much alcohol! A young drinker is then, in the first place, getting to know the crude forces of his astral body. By means of alcohol he can make an impression on others, show his strength, let himself go, etc. But he will also insist that despite many drinks he can still manage to control himself and behave reasonably. The ancient character of alcohol as used in the Mysteries reveals itself once again:

surrendering to the crude force of intoxication and trying to maintain control at the same time.

This is very different from the use of marijuana/hashish at the same stage of life. Marijuana/hashish can be used to let the astral body softly waft away, fuse with the astral body of other users so that the user has more colourful, intense, dreamlike hallucinations and feelings in his own astral body. Alcohol allows the user to experience the strength of the astral body, the power of metabolism in the blood, the power of the ethereal body and of the physical body. Thus, like marijuana, alcohol produces feelings, but they have a coarser, denser more "physical" quality. In this way the astral body – and part of the Self – is linked more strongly to the physical world as stated above, while marijuana/hashish actually allows the astral body to depart to some extent, often after an initial stimulating stage, to fuse with the cosmic astral world.

This is why it is easy to understand why alcohol and marijuana/hashish are the most popular drugs with young people during puberty and adolescence: the newborn astral body is physically bound by alcohol while with marijuana/hashish it separates from the physical world. Both drugs manipulate the astral body, but this happens outside the sphere of the Self. The drugs do the work, taking over the task of the Self. The Self simply stands by and looks on. This inhibits the development of the individual and human qualities, as well as the development of the astral body and the Self.

In examining the effects of alcohol on the user's ethereal body, it should be remembered that, quite apart from the above-mentioned phenomena, alcohol is a toxic substance. This means that the ethereal body partly separates from the physical body because of the effect of the poison. The released ethereal forces penetrate the astral body so that the user is overcome, particularly in the case of high doses. He gradually loses consciousness, and in a sense reverts to being a plant. In this case alcohol has a relaxing effect, removing tension and making the user dozy, sleepy and dreamy. In this sense, it is a narcotic, and it is for that reason that many people have a "nightcap" because the effect of the ethereal forces is to place the astral body in a "sleeping" "vegetative" condition, so that the more relaxed astral body can more easily let go of the physical and ethereal body which feels heavy, particulary if a large dose is taken. The result is that the user falls asleep. This is different from the forceful effect of alcohol, but the drug has also been widely used for a long time for its sleep-inducing effects.

When large doses of alcohol are taken regularly for a long time, the ethereal body can become even further separated from the physical body because of the strong toxic effect. This can result in all sorts of hallucinations and psychotic conditions, such as alcoholic hallucinations and the symptoms which can arise in delirium tremens.

In recent years there have been detailed studies on the effect of alcohol on the user's physical body, and this has been described both in the scientific literature and in layman's literature. Therefore I do not intend to include all this information in detail here, though I will discuss a number of the phenomena in broad terms.

First, there is the well-known hangover which nearly every heavy alcohol user has to cope with the morning after: the symptoms include a splitting headache, nausea, vomiting, dry mouth, poor appetite, irritability, nervousness, shakiness, sweating, easily becoming tired, and a feeling of exhaustion. The hangover is caused by the fact that countless toxic substances have accumulated in the physical body which is exhausted by the alcohol. These include the toxic byproduct of alcohol, acetaldehyde, and increased concentrations of lactic acid, formic acid and uric acid as a result of the metabolic processes of the alcohol. Because of this disruption of the physical body the astral body and the Self will not be able to penetrate the physical body to the same extent when the user awakes and when they "collide" with the physical body again. The astral body and the Self return to the physical body, which has become rather alienated as a result of the effects of alcohol. The user experiences this lack of harmony, this inability to penetrate the physical body which is encumbered with byproducts and waste products, as a painful and unpleasant experience. For a detailed description of a hangover, reference is made to Chapter 6, Opiates, p.115 etc. However in this context it is worth noting that a hangover can be particularly painful in the head, because the metabolism of the brain, which is based on sugar, becomes a sort of process of fermentation (particularly after the use of sweet wines and sweet alcoholic drinks such as port), and this impedes the normal metabolic processes.[71] The result is that the user experiences this lack of harmony combined with the accumulation of toxic substances, as extremely painful.

In addition, there may be withdrawal symptoms after long-term use of medium to high doses, and often also after the occasional use of extreme quantities. These occur when the state of intoxication diminishes, the next day or even later. In this case, the user's physical body has built up a greater or lesser degree of tolerance to alcohol. Therefore fairly permanent defence mechanisms have entered into operation in his physical body, ensuring that the damaging quality of the alcohol is to some extent neutralized. This means that larger doses are necessary to obtain the desired effect – up to a critical point. (However, in the case of a damaged or diseased liver the tolerance declines as the neutralizing function is lost.) This means that it does not cost too much money to stay drunk all the time.

The withdrawal symptoms often take the following form:
— tremors (shaking) of the fingers and tongue;
— psychomotor restlessness, (motor activity) muscular cramps;
— states of confusion, disorientation, disordered thinking;
— sweating, rapid pulse rate, increased blood pressure, raised temperature;
— sleeplessness;
— to a lesser extent, fits, hallucinations, illusions;
— fears and depressive complaints.

These phenomena indicate, in the first place, that the user's astral body and Self are doing their best to re-enter the physical body which is rebelling against the lack of alcohol (increased blood pressure, rapid pulse, psychomotor restlessness, muscular cramps, sweating, insomnia), while his various essential elements have the greatest difficulty in becoming properly reunited with the physical body which is now adapted to an alcoholic metabolism.

This results in a volatile situation:
— After the period of intoxication, the Self and the astral body can no longer find their way "home" to the other parts of the body. They seem to be rejected when they attempt to do so (fits). In this, the low levels of blood sugar also often play a role.
— The Self also has less of a grasp on the thought processes (confusion) and on the restless and powerful involuntary movements of the astral body (psychomotor restlessness).
— The Self, the astral body and the ethereal body can no longer entirely penetrate the limbs of the physical body (tremors and muscular cramps), and the liver, which becomes damaged as a result of the use of alcohol (and other organs such as the brain and the peripheral nervous system).

To summarize, the astral body and the organization of the Self make a huge effort to restore the situation which existed before the start of the alcohol consumption.

If an alcoholic has a few drinks in the morning because of his withdrawal symptoms and the pressing need for alcohol, most of the symptoms rapidly disappear and the unpleasant shakiness will cease. The alcohol has taken possession of him again and he feels "back to normal". The configuration of the various elements of the soul produced by the alcohol has been restored.

In this respect it is understandable that in the past people referred to the alcohol monster, the alcohol demon or the alcohol devil which had taken place of the Self. It was no longer the Self but the alcohol which determined the inter-relationship of the various elements of the soul. In this context Rudolf Steiner also called alcohol the "counter-Self".

Withdrawal symptoms occur in an even more intense form in the case of delirium tremens.[72] This can affect someone who has used alcohol excessively for a long time, when he ends his years of consumption, though it can also occur during a period of excessive consumption. In many cases the physical body has already been injured by the excessive consumption, so that the battle of the other elements of the soul to enter the physical body is greatly intensified. In many cases this is a life and death battle: if they are untreated, about 30% of patients die.[73] An examination of the damage to the user's physical body as a result of long-term excessive consumption reveals that many of the organs are damaged by alcohol.

In the first place, it is well known that the liver suffers greatly from the presence and destructive forces of alcohol. All sorts of metabolic abnormalities occur in the liver and these can eventually lead to complaints and diseases such as degeneration of the liver, hepatitis and finally cirrhosis. In the case of cirrhosis of the liver, the liver cells which have been killed by the alcohol are replaced by connective tissue so that the liver shrinks and the organ can no longer function satisfactorily. Ultimately this results in death.

Thus the ethereal forces leave the liver as a result of alcoholic poisoning. When this happens in a lighter or less serious form it can also lead to complaints of a depressive nature.[74] The user feels that he is lacking in will and seems to be trapped in his past, unable to relate to the future. This fills him with fear and he becomes afraid of life itself. Added to this there are feelings of self-reproach and sometimes sudden outbursts of rage, which can result in suicide.

The heart is also involved in the depression caused by damage to the liver. R. Treichler wrote: "The link with the heart is an essential aspect of this depression. The fact that the heart is affected is revealed by the compulsive organic feelings of guilt, i.e. the self-reproach of the Self. This can assume the dimensions of a delusion: "I am the worst housewife that has ever lived; my life is worth nothing".[75] Many alcoholics will recognize these feelings.

Moreover, after many years of extreme alcoholic consumption, an alcohol-induced hallucinogenic state can arise as a result of the partially lost ethereal forces. The user suffers from massive aural hallucinations which often threaten him and therefore fill him with terror (for the connection between the liver and LSD hallucinations, see pp. 61–63). In addition, there can be damage to the gastrointestinal system (haemorrhaging in the stomach, ulcers, cancer of the oesophagus) and to the kidneys and adrenal glands. Furthermore, the pancreas (pancreatic tissue is replaced by connective tissue) and the thyroid gland are often damaged. The hormonal system becomes confused. Alcoholics often have a lower level of male hormones (testosterone) and an increased level of the female sexual hormones in the blood (this can often be demonstrated when there is liver damage).[76] This results in the body becoming more "feminine", with symptoms such as withered testicles, the development of breasts and a loss of pubic hair.[77] In addition, there may be general muscular weakness during periods of excessive drinking when the tissue in the muscles atrophies. Furthermore, the alcoholic's resistance to infection is greatly reduced.

There are far reaching consequences for reproduction:

a.   In half of chronic users of alcohol there is a loss of libido – often in addition to the symptoms described above – which is frequently accompanied by abnormalities in the semen as a result of damage to the seminal tube. "After abstaining from alcohol the libido and sexual potency recover very slowly and then only if the alcoholic's testicles have not atrophied and have a normal sperm concentration".[78] "The sperm abnormalities of chronic alcoholics are often (25%) irreversible, even after they stop drinking alcohol, though there is some reversal in most men after about eight weeks."[76] It is difficult to ascertain the consequences for the offspring of humans objectively. However, tests on animals have shown that "the rats from nests in which the fathers have been fed with alcohol were significantly smaller and lighter and presented different behaviour from their siblings from a control group. Furthermore, the number of nests and the number of rats per nest were smaller than in the control group."[79]

In 50% of women who drink more than 3 glasses of alcohol per day there are abnormalities in the menstrual cycle. In most of them there are also changes in the hormone system (lower levels of oestrogen and progesterone).[80] In addition, there are frequent miscarriages and infertility.[81]

b. There is also the so-called foetal alcohol syndrome (FAS), described by Jones in 1973, which means that children of female alcoholics can develop a fixed pattern of prenatal and postnatal physical abnormalities, such as:
- retarded growth;
- low birth weight;
- small circumference of the skull, brain abnormalities, abnormalities of the central nervous system resulting in neurological, intellectual and/or behaviourial problems;
- abnormal appearance, low hair line (very small forehead), short gap between the eyelids, flat nose, distorted external ear, insufficiently developed upper jaw, small thin upper lip without a groove or with a flattened groove; the *human* countenance becomes deformed:
- abnormalities of the limbs, reduced mobility of the joints, short nails, the lines of the hand are different, heart (valve) defects, kidney defects, abnormalities of the female sexual organs.

Some additional facts:
- These abnormalities never occur altogether in one child.
- The cause probably lies in the effect of the alcohol or acetaldehyde during the period just before and during the first three months of pregnancy, while drinking during the second half of pregnancy can result in retarded growth and can result in brain damage.[82]
- "The tremors, nervous frightened behaviour, the restlessness in the rhythm of sleeping and waking, and the excessive reflex activity of FAS babies are based on the abnormal arrangement of the organs."[83]
- In his book, *Alcoholism*, R. Spieksma wrote: "Various sources have shown that drinking alcohol during the earlier stages of pregnancy can result in the birth of children with defects which indicate FAS. Most women are not even aware at this stage that they are pregnant (a few days late); even a small quantity of alcohol (such as 3 to 4 glasses of wine per day) or a single occasion of heavy drinking results in significant differences when compared with a control group. This is not a question of female alcoholics, but of

ordinary social drinkers. Social drinking during later stages of pregnancy entails fewer risks for the foetus, because the placenta has already been formed (acetaldehyde is broken down in the placenta so that no more acetaldehyde is found in the foetus after the sixteenth week when the placenta has been formed). However, there are more still births because the placenta can become detached, even when only 3 or 4 glasses are drunk per day".[84]

— "Therefore it is always advisable for women who wish to become pregnant not to drink a drop of alcohol. Celebrating the pregnancy with a bottle of champagne is therefore out of the question!"[85]

In addition, alcohol enters the marrow in the bones where the blood is formed (the white and red corpuscles). Alcohol has a direct inhibiting effect on the bone marrow; less blood is made.[86]

Van Epen wrote: "Alcoholism leads to different forms of anaemia while the formation of blood platelets necessary for the clotting mechanism, can also be affected."[87]

In addition, there may be disorders in the cardiac and vascular system, such as damage to the cardiac muscle (often as a result of vitamin deficiency – lack of thiamin). The so-called "holiday heart" (abnormalities in cardiac rhythm, enlargement of the heart, oedema etc. as a result of extreme alcoholic consumption on holiday, at the weekend, at parties etc.), and increased blood pressure in the case of more than three drinks per day.

However, recent research shows that the use of alcohol can also have a "protective effect on the development of coronary sclerosis (the furring up of the coronary arteries) resulting in angina pectoris and eventually leading to heart attacks)".[88]

Half of chronic alcoholics show signs of having damaged nerves in the arms and legs. After a time this can result in abnormalities in the sensory system and even paralysis; examination reveals that the reflexes have disappeared. This nervous condition is caused mainly by the vitamin B deficiency (thiamin).[89]

Long-term excessive alcohol consumption can result in serious brain damage (particularly as a result of a vitamin B1 deficiency); "The most important symptom is premature dementia, which can vary from memory loss to the serious Wernicke-Korsakoff syndrome".[90] In the latter case there is a reduction in the capacity to concentrate, short-term memory loss and problems with walking (the Self is forced to withdraw from the disordered organization of the Self). At a later stage the memory loss increases leading to so-called confabulations (untrue fantasies not controlled by the Self). This is followed by a confusion with regard to the experience of time, space and place (the ethereal body also partly retreats from the damaged brain). The alcoholic no longer recognizes people from his direct social environment and ultimately he may suffer from dementia even at a young age. Van Epen wrote: "As a result of the increase in alcoholism there is also an increase in the number of chronic, incurable Korsakoff patients. They are admitted to permanent wards in psychiatric hospitals or other special provisions are made".[91]

I can conclude that during the state of intoxication the Self is expelled to a greater or lesser extent as a result of the partial disintegration of the organization of the Self. This produces a pleasant, light and liberated feeling. Cares, problems and loneliness disappear and seem to dissolve in the comfortable warmth of the "consoler" which grants oblivion.

However, the astral forces (which are connected to the body) now have their chance instead of the Self. They give the uninhibited user a sense of power, while at the same time the ethereal and physical forces of the Self – insofar as they are still present – connect with these influences coming "from below". The Self is found at the level of the animal, vegetative state (which is intoxicated and repeats itself) and of the physical state (which is rigid and heavy).

In this way alcohol separates man from his own essence, from his own Self and from his own unique identity.

The chronic consumption of alcohol chains man to the earth allowing his astral body to manifest itself as a sort of pseudo-Self while man repeats himself and his physical body starts to fall apart.

8

Cocaine and amphetamines

Cocaine

History

When the first European explorers landed in South America at the beginning of the 16th century they discovered a strange custom among the local population. In a letter dated 7 September 1504, Amerigo Vespucci wrote: "They were very ugly in appearance and in their habits. They all puffed up their cheeks with a green herb on which they chewed constantly like cows. They could hardly speak and they all wore two gourds around their neck. One was full of the herb which everyone had in their mouth, the other was full of a white flour that looked rather like plaster. From time to time they would moisten a stick, put it in the flour and place it in their mouths ... In this way they mixed the flour with the herb ... and because we were very surprised by this we could not understand the secret."[1]

The Conquistadors had never come across this phenomenon of chewing the leaves of the coca bush in combination with some chalk or a powder made of crushed shells to facilitate the release of cocaine from the leaves. This was entirely unknown in European culture. However, for the Indians of South America this custom had a very long history which can be summarized as follows.

The first signs which indicate the use of coca were discovered along the coast of Ecuador. These include illustrations of people chewing coca leaves which have been dated approximately 3000 BC. From Ecuador the custom spread to the coast of Peru where well-conserved coca leaves dating from approximately 1300 BC have been found, and then spread over the whole of the South American continent. Many archaeological discoveries revealed that the priests and shamans used the drug in their religious and medicinal activities.

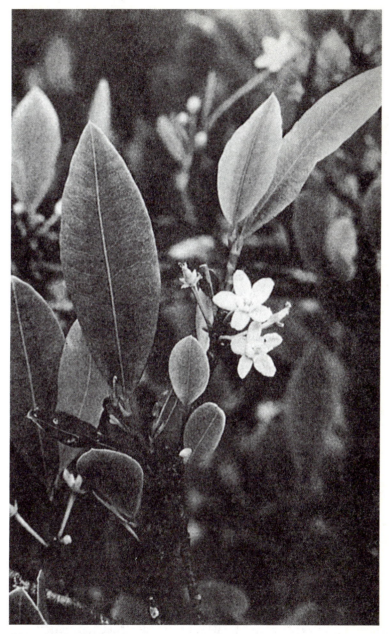

Photograph: A flowering branch of Columbian coca in Peru.

During the time of the Incas (1020–1533 AD) the cultivation and dissemination of the coca plant increased and became more widespread. For the Incas, coca was a sacred plant which had come to them from the world of the gods. According to the myth, Manco Capac, the divine son of the Sun, had descended from the rocks near Lake Titicaca in the dim and distant past to bring knowledge to mankind: he brought the poor dwellers of the earth the light of his father, taught them to know the gods, instructed them in useful arts, and gave them coca "the divine plant which satisfies the hungry, gives strength to the weak and helps man to forget adversity."[2]

Nevertheless, the use of coca was initially restricted to the caste of priests and the chosen nobility though they could give their permission to other people to use this drug in exceptional cases.

Coca played a role in religious rituals, initiation ceremonies and sometimes on special occasions. Some examples are given below:
- Offerings of coca leaves were made during certain ceremonies; the priests predicted the future from the smoke of the burning leaves. Those who submitted petitions could only approach the altar if they had coca leaves in their mouths.
- During the "Huraca", the initiation ceremony for young noblemen, races were held and young girls gave the runners coca as they ran. At the finish, every participant would be given a "chuspa" (shoulder bag) filled with coca leaves as the sign that he had proved his masculinity.
- Men who were responsible for storing important facts in their memory (as there were no adequate written records for this purpose), were permitted to chew coca to strengthen their powers of recall.
- In religious rituals coca leaves were burned in the temple like incense; the images of the gods carried the coca leaves in their hands.

All these examples show that coca played a very important role in Inca culture, and therefore it is not surprising that the use of this drug gradually started to spread amongst larger and larger groups of the population.

When Pisarro conquered the Inca empire with his 180 Conquistadors in 1533, the use of coca had become commonplace among a large section of the population, although chewing coca still had a religious significance.

For the Christian Spaniards who entered the former Inca empire in ever greater numbers, this use of coca was rather enigmatic. They tried to understand it: "When you ask the Indians why they always have their mouths full of those herbs which they do not eat but merely keep between their teeth, they say that it makes them feel less hungry, stronger and more powerful. I think it must have that sort of effect, although it seems a sin or a bad habit which seems to suit people like these Indians." (Pedro Ciezo de Leon at the beginning of the 16th century).[3]

Gradually, opinions about this habit became more negative. The magic of chewing coca was seen as the main obstacle to the conversion of the Indians to Christianity, and during the First Church Council in Lima in 1551 (and also in 1567) coca was prohibited: "A useless, dissolute thing which leads to superstition and temptation by the devil."[4] Other writers from that time wrote: "Coca was discovered by the devil for the complete destruction of the natives." (Diego de Robiez)[5] and "Coca is an important element in the service of idolatry, the Indian's ceremonies and witchcraft, and their insistence that when they have it in their mouth they have power is an intimation of the devil, as experienced people say" (the King of Spain in a decree dated 1569).[6]

Prohibitions were passed on the cult, chewing and cultivation of coca, and penalties were imposed for the violations of these prohibitions, but this did not help much. On 15 July 1579, the Catholic priest, Antonio de Zunida, wrote in a letter to the Spanish king that he had not succeeded in converting the heathens because of their habit of using coca, and he argued for much harsher measures: the destruction of all the coca plantations and the sale of all the Indians who had worked on the plantations as slaves.

However, this did not happen. The Spanish started to realize that the use of coca could not be eradicated, because the roots of this custom were too deep in the centuries-old culture. Moreover, it provided opportunities in the form of hard-working labourers who required little food, thus resulting in higher profits. While the Spanish were still in power, the prohibitions were lifted. It was accepted that Indians needed coca so that they could perform their heavy work, for example, in the gold and silver mines, often in extreme conditions (cold, great heights and so on).

The trade in coca started to flourish. Coca leaves were even used as a form of currency and, at the end of the 16th century, a regular coca industry had developed employing about 2,000 Spaniards. The profits were enormous, more or less comparable with the profits of the gold and silver mines.

In their turn, the Indians integrated their ancient myths in the Christianity that was foisted upon them, resulting for example, in the myth of "Mama Coca", the story of the Virgin Mary who lay down to rest under a tree during her flight from Egypt. Sunk in dreams she had tasted the leaves of this tree. As soon as she had chewed these just a little,she had felt refreshed and strengthened."[5] This tale merely confirmed the sacred nature of coca for the Indians.

Towards the end of the 16th and beginning of the 17th century the use of coca was a completely accepted phenomenon in and near the Andes. Some of the white colonists had even taken up the habit. Furthermore, the Spanish had discovered that coca could be used as an important medicine. For example, the Jesuit priest, Bernabe Cobo, described how the Indians had taught him to use coca leaves for broken bones and infected wounds, and for cases of indigestion, or to administer them for severe vomiting.

Scientific researchers and traders travelling through the Andes in the 19th century discovered that the use of coca was widespread. Some of them tried it themselves, like Clement Markham who visited Peru in 1859: "I chewed Coca, not constantly but frequently ... and besides the agreeable soothing feeling it produced, I found that I could endure long abstinence from food with less inconvenience than I should otherwise have felt, and it enabled me to ascend precipitous mountain sides with a feeling of lightness and elasticity and without losing breath. This latter quality ought to recommend its use to members of the Alpine Club, and to walking tourists in general."[7]

To this very day coca plays an extremely important role in the Indian culture in and around the Andes region and in the jungles of the Amazon basin. Coca is used in religious rituals in soothsaying and medicine, and helps the Indians to do their heavy work in the mines, often at great heights. It actually increases the heart's activity and speeds up respiration, so that the body has a better supply of oxygen at great heights. It is used in various ways in medicine to anaesthetize all sorts of aches and pains such as headaches, infected wounds, stomach aches, labour pains and so on. Coca is also used in social intercourse: when two friends meet they often make each other a gift of coco leaves as a sign of welcome, just as we offer a guest a cup of coffee, tea or a glass of wine.

The number of coqueros – as the Indians call the users – is estimated to be more than eight million people, mostly men. It is assumed that 90% of men chew coca to a greater or lesser extent.[8] The amount of pure cocaine which a chronic user would consume every day in this way is estimated to be between 0.14[9] and 0.5 grammes.[10] In comparison with an addict who sniffs or injects cocaine, this is between a low and comparable dose. However, because of the lengthy chewing process (approximately 40 minutes) and the fact that the cocaine is diluted with saliva, it has a less rapid and less intense effect than injecting or sniffing it, when the much purer cocaine enters the blood considerably faster or almost directly.

As regards the consequences for Indians, there are various opinions from "a statistical correlation between illiteracy and coca-chewing, between lack of interest and reduced aptitude in learning and coca-chewing, and between malnutrition and coca-chewing",[11] to: "the risks of chewing coca are comparable to the risks of drinking coffee and tea."[12]

However, the use of coca gives Indians an important sense of their own value. Ganzer et al. wrote: "Coca was and is still a psychological and physical aid for Indians to help them escape from the most serious suppression and terrible circumstances. Coca is something which belongs to them. The communal use of this drug, whether it is in a ritual cult or as a medicine, gives them a sense of belonging and power."[13]

Before we continue with a description of the history of cocaine in Europe, we will briefly examine the plant from which cocaine is derived.

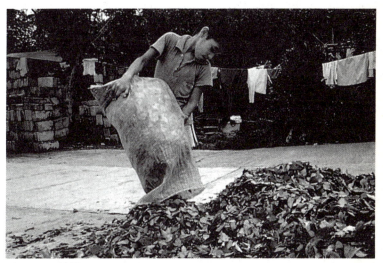

Photograph: Harvesting the coca leaves.

The coca plant

The coca plant is a shrub which is several metres tall and which grows in the Andes mountains at heights between 500 and 2,000 metres. In the wild the plant can grow to a height of 5 metres, but to facilitate the harvest of the leaves, the shrubs are pruned to a height of 1–2 metres. The plant flowers with yellowish flowers; the fruits are rock hard and red. The leaves, for which the plant is grown, are delicate, lanceolate, and abundant. They are harvested three or four times a year (see photograph on p.203). They contain the highest concentration of cocaine at an average daytime temperature of 15°C (during the growing and ripening period). The coca plant thrives best in humid, warm mountainous regions and is grown there on small terraced areas. In the past coca plantations were found not only in the Andes but also in Java, Sri Lanka, India, Africa and in the West Indian Archipelago. However, it is now cultivated solely in the South American continent.

Cocaine in Europe

In 1569, the first coca leaves were imported into Europe. The coca plant itself was not imported until 1749. At first little attention was paid to either. In 1783, Jean Baptiste Lamarck successfully classified the plant in the class Erythroxylaceae, and from that time it was called: *Erythroxylon coca* (Lamarck). It was only in the 19th century that the reports of famous explorers and scientists, such as Alexander von Humbolt and Eduard Poeppig, came to the ears of the European public and scientific circles. The coca leaves which they brought home with them were studied in scientific institutes to discover their "secret" powers.

In 1860 (possibly even in 1859), Alfred Niemann successfully isolated the most important active ingredient of the coca leaf: this was the alkaloid, methyl-benzoyl-ecgonine, which he called cocaine. More or less at the same time (1859) the first complete European book on coca was published. It was written by the Italian anthropologist-doctor, and writer of novels and fairy tales, Paolo Mantegazza, who described the use of coca as a positive thing on the basis of his own experience: "Borne by two wing-like coca leaves I flew through 77,348 worlds, one more beautiful than the next. God is unjust because he has organized things in such a way that man can live without constantly chewing coca. I would prefer a life with coca above a life of a million centuries without coca."[14]

In the 1860s the production, trade and sale of cocaine flourished. In southern Europe the drug was particularly popular as a stimulant, while it also gained popularity in central and northern Europe, first as a medicine, and later as a stimulant. In 1863, wine containing cocaine appeared on the market: this was the "strengthening elixir", Vin Mariani, produced by the French pharmacist, Angelo Mariani. Many famous people from that time praised it profusely in his yearbook after taking it themselves. These included the writers, Emile Zola, Jules Verne and Henrik Ibsen, the composers, Charles Gounod, Jules Massenet and John Sousa, the painter, Mucha, and the inventor, Thomas Edison. Czar Alexander II and Pope Leo XIII are also known to have drunk the elixir.

Coca wines, coca champagnes, coca pastilles and coca cigarettes appeared everywhere in Europe. To give just one impression (1881): "I would also like to say that in virtually all pharmacies in Paris, coca specialities and coca wine are prepared on medical prescription. Coca leaves are sold in all the pharmacies in Paris. They can also be found in the larger pharmacies in Italy ... All the cafés in Italy serve the Elixir de Coca Boliviana, produced by a large company which has specialised in this product."[15]

Coca Cola

In 1886, John Styth Pemperton introduced Coca Cola onto the market. This was an alcohol-free syrup which contained cocaine and was initially recommended particularly for its medicinal properties. One of the first advertisements from that time was: "Coca cola is not only a delicious, refreshing, reviving and fortifying drink" , but also a valuable "food for the brain which can cure all sorts of nervous symptoms, such as nervous headaches, neuralgia, hysteria and melancholy."[16]

Pemberton had chosen the right time; in some of the American states alcohol had been prohibited by the radical Temperance Movement, and therefore Coca Cola proved to be an excellent alternative. Two years after it was introduced, the medical allusions disappeared from the advertisements and henceforth Coca Cola was advertised as a "refreshing and reviving drink."[16] However, when the radical movement opposing drink and addiction discovered the dangers of cocaine (following negative publications on cocaine as a problem drug) the Coca Cola company was put under great pressure to remove the cocaine from the drink and, in 1903, the cocaine was replaced by caffeine.

However, to this very day the leaves of the coca plant are still used as one of the ingredients. They give the Coca Cola its special smell though they are "de-cocainized" (the cocaine is extracted).

The end of the 19th century

During the last decade of the 19th century cocaine was scientifically investigated and used in a number of different ways:

- From the beginning of the 1880s the drug played a supportive role – particularly in the United States – in helping alcoholics and morphine addicts to kick their habits (as a substitute). However, when increasingly negative reports on the harmful effects of cocaine appeared in the medical press during the 1890s, cocaine gradually lost this function, and from 1898 it was replaced by the new and promising substitute: heroin, for the treatment of morphine addicts.

- A great deal of research was carried out in the medical world into the medical applications of cocaine. It was used amongst other things as a medicine for colds and 'flu, as a restorative remedy to counteract the consequences of a sedentary life style, and as a general remedy for digestive disorders and migraines. Cocaine factories were established in several other countries; the "Dutch Cocaine Factory" was founded in about 1870. This factory produced medicines with a cocaine base.

The Viennese eye specialist, Carl Koller, was the first to discover the properties of cocaine for use as a local anaesthetic, following earlier observations and research by Karl Schroff in 1862 and Von Anrep in 1879. He recounted the following anecdote: "Doctor Engel took a little bit of cocaine on the tip of his pocket knife and said: "How that numbs the tongue!", I said: "Yes, everyone who has tried to eat it has noticed that", at that moment I suddenly realized that I was carrying in my pocket the local anaesthetic which I had been looking for for years."[17]

First of all, Koller tried out cocaine on frogs and then on warm-blooded animals. Subsequently, when these experiments proved to be successful, he used cocaine as a local anaesthetic when he performed eye operations on his patients. This was extremely significant. Alfred Springer wrote: "It is only possible to appreciate the importance of this step when you imagine the infinite pain which people had to suffer up to that time when they underwent an operation on the eye."[18] Cocaine made it possible to perform operations on the eye which had been impossible up to that time.

On 15 September 1884, Koller presented his discovery during a conference with medical colleagues in Heidelberg. From that time cocaine was extremely popular as the single best local anaesthetic and was used not only for operations on the eyes but also for operations on the nose, throat, ears, etc. Cocaine is used for this reason up to this very day, even though there are many other substances now which have a comparable effect such as novocaine, scandicaine, xylocaine, lidocaine and others.

– The group of researchers who experimented with cocaine in Vienna included Sigmund Freud as well as Carl Koller. From 1884 to 1887 he performed many experiments on himself. Initially he was enormously enthusiastic (see his letter to his fiancée dated 2 April 1884, which is quoted on p. 33). He was encouraged to carry out scientific research so that he could write "an ode to this miracle drug." In his next letter (21 April 1884) the 28-year-old Freud wrote to her: "I am now working on a promising project and I would like to tell you about it, but perhaps nothing will come of it." "It is a therapeutic experiment. I am reading about cocaine, the active ingredient of coca leaves which many Indian tribes chew so that they can tolerate hardship and great exertion. A German has tried this substance on soldiers and found that it does have a wonderfully strengthening effect and can increase a person's performance. I would like to obtain some of this, and for obvious reasons I would like to try it out in cases of heart disease and also for nervous conditions, particularly for curing morphine addiction (as in Doctor Fleischl). Perhaps many others are working on it and perhaps it is no good. But I certainly want to try it out, and you know that if you try often enough and want to succeed, you will be successful one day."[19]

A few months later he published the results of his study in *Uber Coca*. A subsequent study, in which he was assisted by Carl Koller, was published in January 1885 with the title: *A Contribution to the Knowledge about the Effects of Coca*. Several other articles followed.

In *Uber Coca*, Freud already recommended the substance for the treatment of the most diverse "psychological conditions" such as "hysteria, hypochondria, melancholia, stupor and so on."[20] He also recommended cocaine for neurasthenia, asthma, digestive disorders and psychological impotence. As regards the latter, he describes the case of a writer who "was unable to produce any literature for weeks, but was able to work for 14 hours without interruption after taking cocaine."[20] During these years he also performed experiments on himself which he described in great detail: " I have experienced this effect of coca which provides protection against hunger, sleep and fatigue and stimulates mental work, about a dozen times."[21] After a while he also started to use small doses of cocaine as a medicine to relieve his (slight) neurotic complaint.

The change came when his very good friend, Doctor Fleischl, for whom he had prescribed cocaine to cure his morphine addiction, became addicted to cocaine after a while. Jürgen vom Scheidt wrote: "In May 1884 he prescribed the alkaloid for his friend, Ernst von Fleischl-Marxow and cured him, as he still thought in 1887, of his morphine addiction. A few years later he realized to his enormous dismay that he had merely led his friend to a new addiction and had hastened his end."[22] When Fleischl died in 1891, partly as a result of his excessive doses of cocaine, this probably also meant the end of Freud's cocaine consumption;[23] though it was still prescribed for him temporarily in 1895 as a medicine against a "swelling in the nose."

Others have emphasized that Freud had already stopped using cocaine in 1887 because he was in danger of becoming professionally and scientifically isolated as a result of his enthusiasm for the drug. From 1886 there were many articles in the press recording cases of cocaine poisoning and cocaine addiction, with the result that the scientific world resolutely turned against the consumption of cocaine as a stimulant and as a medicine. Freud defended himself against his critics in *On Cocaine Addiction and the Fear of Cocaine* (1887). Later in *The Interpretation of Dreams* (1889), he wrote that: "His recommendation of cocaine had resulted in serious allegations against him in Vienna."[24]

The 20th Century

The first article about a new way of taking cocaine appeared in 1900 in *The Journal of the American Medical Association*. This concerned sniffing cocaine: "The Negroes in some parts of the South are reported as being addicted to a new form of vice – that of cocaine 'snuffing' or the 'coke habit'!"[25] A few years later, this use of cocaine was also experimented with in Europe, particularly in Paris, amongst artists and intellectuals (there was already a tradition of the use of hashish in Paris – "the Club des Haschischins" – dating from the previous century), and "the dregs of society, the irresponsible, liars, swindlers and enemies of society", as problem groups were known at the time (survey in 1913).[26]

During the First World War, cocaine was used by pilots: "Many French and German pilots filled their nostrils with white powder ('snow') before they took off into the air."[23]

After the First World War, particularly during the 1920s, which were known as the "Roaring Twenties", cocaine became extremely popular in many large European cities. There was a trade in cocaine which came onto the market after the First World War. The extremely insecure and revolutionary social and economic situation with gigantic inflation provided an ideal basis for this drug which resulted in temporary euphoria. In 1921, the Italian Futurist, F.T. Marinetti, characterized the atmosphere of that time as follows: "The coarse and primitive majority of mankind throw themselves tempestuously at the revolutionary conquest of the communist paradise and at the final victory of happiness, with the firm conviction that all needs and material desires can be satisfactorily assuaged. The intellectual minority ironically despises this exhausting attempt, sees life as a cruel process and surrenders to a feeble pessimism, sexual perversions and the artificial paradise of cocaine, opium, ether ... as the former joys of religion, art and love which were once their privilege and escape, are no longer in vogue."[27]

A song from Berlin at that time describes this mood amongst the young as follows:

> And therefore, we from Berlin
> Grab cocaine and morphine,
> Even though thunder and lightning rage outside,
> We sniff and we shoot up! ...
> Therefore, when we are tortured by worry,
> We sniff and we shoot up!

And it ended:

> And if you shoot your way into the madhouse
> And if you sniff your way to death –
> Dear God, what does it matter
> At this time and in this world?
> Europe is a madhouse anyway
> And today one would like to creep

Above all into paradise
By sniffing and shooting up.[28]

In America a great deal of cocaine was used in the 1920s; there it was part of an atmosphere of optimism, money, freedom and so on. This was very different from the attitude in Europe. In the 1930s, which saw the economic depression, the use of cocaine in America dropped significantly to be replaced by marijuana and, from 1933, by alcohol which had once again been legalized.

In Europe, the use of cocaine also declined in the 1930s; by the outbreak of the Second World War it had dwindled to a negligible phenomenon.

After the Second World War

During and after the Second World War there was very little evidence of cocaine being used for non-medical purposes; the stimulants which were used on a large scale at that time by soldiers and later by millions of Japanese and many Scandinavians, were entirely synthetic and belonged to the group of so-called "wekamins" such as amphetamines.

Cocaine reappeared in the United States only at the end of the 1970s, where it found a fertile climate because the disadvantages and dangers of the purely synthetic stimulants (speed) had been discovered by many users. Cocaine seemed to be far less harmful; after all, it was derived from natural raw materials, and the Indians had been chewing on coca leaves for thousands of years. The lessons of the 1920s, and the tens of thousands of cocaine addicts, had been forgotten.[29]

The great breakthrough for cocaine took place in the 1980s, the "no nonsense" era when the expensive drug was increasingly used by people in the film, music and media world, and by yuppies, drug addicts and so on.

In the mid-1980s the drug was "democratized": a much cheaper, stronger variation appeared on the American market. This was "crack." (Crack is cocaine which is boiled with sodium bicarbonate or bicarbonate of soda and water. When it cools down there is a sediment which is broken into pieces or "rocks." These rocks can be smoked.) Crack has an extremely powerful and short-lived effect (3-5 minutes); the kick is incredibly euphoric, and while the user is under the influence she feels that she can confront the whole world, both physically and psychologically, in an extremely aggressive way.

Furthermore, it has the advantage that it can be smoked, so that the effect is felt after only a few seconds, unlike cocaine which is generally sniffed and only reaches the brain after several minutes via the mucous membrane in the nose and the blood. Crack leads to addiction very quickly and has led to an increase in the number of cocaine or crack users in the United States to an estimated 22 million people.

However, the wave of crack in the United States has up to now hardly reached Europe, though the "cocaine bases" introduced from Surinam have been used in the Netherlands since about the mid-1980s. For this, cocaine is mixed with bicarbonate of soda through a water pipe, generally filled with rum, and smoked. As a result the cocaine quickly reaches the blood mixed with alcohol vapour and is often accompanied by outbursts of extreme aggression.[30]

Nowadays, the illegal production, trade and sale of cocaine has become an extremely lucrative business. The tens of millions of users and addicts, particularly in the United States and Europe, are supplied by mafiosi drug cartels from Bolivia, Peru, Ecuador and so on, who run the trade. The profits from these cartels are enormous despite the American "war on drugs", particularly because of the growing markets in Europe (especially Eastern Europe). In the late 1970s, early 1980s, it is estimated that the illegal turnover of marijuana/hashish was approximately just as high as the turnover of the world oil industry. Since then, cocaine, which is much more expensive, has partly taken the place of marijuana/hashish and has grown to epidemic proportions. The profits of the cocaine mafiosi have undoubtedly risen to unimaginable levels.[31]

The effects of cocaine

As described in the section on the history of cocaine, this drug has an anaesthetizing, stimulating and euphoric effect. We will discuss these different effects below, once again looking in particular at the effect of cocaine on the different parts of the human soul.

The anaesthetizing effect

Cocaine has an anaesthetizing effect on the central nervous system, and particularly on the peripheral nervous system, by blocking the conduction of stimuli by the sensory nerves. For example, if the drug reaches the mucous membranes of the stomach wall, feelings of hunger and thirst are dulled, as we saw in the discussion on the chewing of coca leaves by the Indians.

Here are a few other examples, apart from the local anaesthetizing effect discussed above:
— When a low dose of cocaine is injected into the spinal cord, all the parts of the body below the waist are anaesthetized and can be operated on.[32]
— When cocaine gets into the blood by being smoked, sniffed or being injected, the drug has an anaesthetizing effect on certain ganglia of the nervous system rendering them insensitive to stimuli.[33]

The above shows that consciousness, i.e. the astral body, withdraws from the parts of the nervous system taken over by cocaine; part of the astral body separates, as though it is breathed out. (In the case of an extremely low dose this means that the user falls into a quiet, more relaxed dreamy and sleepy state; in addition, the heartbeat slows down.)

On the other hand, the astral body also "breathes in" (when a higher dose is taken) so that this results in increased stimulation and alertness.

The stimulant effect

The reinforced effect of the astral body can be seen in a large number of symptoms:
— increased rate of respiration (though it is no deeper);
— a high dose can result in very rapid superficial respiration;
— an increased heartbeat, at least in the case of normal and high doses; also an increase in blood pressure as the result of the constriction of the peripheral capillaries;
— a slight increase in body temperature; in animals (horses and dogs) the temperature can rise by as much as 3°C;
— stimulation of certain parts of the brain,[34] and in addition, the sympathetic part of the vegetative nervous system, with the result that the pupils dilate;
— an increase in intestinal movements; cocaine has a laxative effect; in addition, the bladder is stimulated resulting in frequent urination;
— a temporary increase in energy and stamina; an increase in restlessness – the user wants to be active.

It is as though the strong "breathing in" of the astral body makes the user extra alert. Tiredness and the desire to sleep disappear and are overridden by the strong, descending astral forces. The astral body is all-powerful, the user seems to "glow" and "sparkle" in his stimulated, almost exhibitionist astral body. Feelings of vulnerability, doubt, insecurity and fear are overwhelmed by this surfeit of astral forces. The emotional reactions are therefore often unusually violent and can easily turn into aggressive outbursts. Sexual desire is stimulated. Jürgen vom Scheidt wrote: "There is a very quick feeling of enormous energy, accompanied by the will to act or talk. The libido is also stimulated, particularly during the first high."[35]

The increase in stamina, i.e. physical performance, is also very striking. The strongly "breathed in" astral body does not allow for feelings of tiredness and exhaustion, with the result that while she is under the effect of the drug, the user feels wide awake, powerful and full of vitality.

- Freud remarked: "You notice ... that you are full of vitality and the will to work ... you can perform long and intense mental or physical tasks without a trace of fatigue."[36]
- The Swedish ethnographer, Erland Nordenskiöld wrote that his Indian guide could carry up to 30 kilos of luggage for 17 hours walking through the mountains. "Without coca, this would be impossible."[37]
- "The Indians can march long distances through the mountains without feeling hungry or exhausted. The 'Cocade' has become a unit of distance, viz., the distance which can be travelled with a certain dose of coca leaves (just like our farmers used to measure the distance between two villages in the number of pipes of tobacco they could smoke on the way)."[38]
- Frank, aged 21, wrote: "When I went to a disco I would be hanging on the bar, exhausted by two o'clock, so I would go to the toilet, sniff some cocaine and come back wide awake. That way you could go on until at least six o' clock."[39] "No wonder that in extremely competitive races and sports, such as the Tour de France or the Berlin Six Day Race, cocaine was sometimes used as a drug (before the modern amphetamines appeared)."[37]

The euphoria

This tremendous "breathing in" of the astral body gives the user a wonderful feeling. Her sense of her own value increases and she feels that she can tackle the whole world. She is speedy, hard and self-assured, does not feel any fear and dares to do anything. "Young, speedy, wild – that's what you wanna be!" This advertisement for Radio Veronica could almost be an advertisement for cocaine.

Cocaine also stimulates the thought processes. The head feels hyperactive; it is light and bright, and associations are made with lightning speed. A few examples are given below:

– "The user ... has the feeling that he can make sharper judgements and think more clearly."[40]
– "Cocaine ... gives you the sense of being able to think exceptionally quickly and clearly."[41]
– "Your own thoughts are experienced as being extremely clear ... For a short time the user feels intensely happy."[42]
– Sherlock Holmes also enjoyed this. In Sir Arthur Conan Doyle's story, *The Sign of Four*, Dr. Watson says: "Sherlock Holmes took his bottle from the corner of the mantlepiece, and his hypodermic syringe from its neat morocco case. With his long, white nervous fingers he adjusted the delicate needle, and rolled back his left shirt-cuff. For some little time his eyes rested thoughtfully upon the sinewy forearm and wrist, all dotted and scarred with innumerable puncture-marks. Finally, he thrust the sharp point home, pressed down the tiny piston and sank back into the velvet-lined armchair with a long sigh of satisfaction.

"Three times a day for many months I had witnessed this performance, but the custom had not reconciled my mind to it. On the contrary, from day to day I had become more irritable at the sight, as my conscience swelled nightly within me at the thought that I had lacked the courage to protest. Again and again I had registered a vow that I should deliver my soul upon the subject; but there was that in the cool, nonchalant air of my companion which made him the last man with whom one would care to take anything approaching to a liberty.

" ... I suddenly felt that I could hold out no longer.

"'Which is it today I asked, morphine or cocaine?'

"He raised his eyes languidly from the old black-letter volume which he had opened.

"'It is cocaine, a seven-per-cent solution. Would you care to try it?'

"'No, indeed,' I answered brusquely ...

"He smiled at my vehemence. 'Perhaps you are right, Watson', he said, 'I suppose that its influence is physically a bad one. I find it, however, so transcendingly stimulating and clarifying to the mind that its second action is a matter of small moment.'

"'But consider!' I said, earnestly. 'Count the loss! Your brain may, as you say, be roused and excited, but it is a pathological and morbid process, which involves increased tissue-change, and may at last leave a permanent weakness. You know, too, what a black reaction comes upon you. Surely the game is hardly worth the candle. Why should you, for a mere passing pleasure, risk the loss of those great powers with which you have been endowed. Remember that I speak not only as one comrade to another, but as a medical man to one for whose constitution he is to some extent answerable.'

"He did not seem offended. On the contrary, he put his fingertips together, and leaned his elbows on the arms of his chair, like one who has a relish for conversation.

"'My mind,' he said, 'rebels at stagnation. Give me problems, give me work, give me the most abstruse cryptogram or the most intricate analysis, and I am in my own proper atmosphere. I can dispense then with artificial stimulants. I crave for mental exultation. That is why I have chosen my own particular profession, or rather created it, for I am the only one in the world'."[43]

Even Sherlock Holmes does not seem to have escaped the feeling of superiority produced by cocaine!

Thus, cocaine results in experiences of "mental stimulation", great clarity and rapidity of thought. In this way the user enters a light, bright world of accelerated associations, which gives her the feeling of being capable of great intellectual and creative achievements, though these often prove to be based on an illusion, because the drug is not objectively able to increase the capacity for thought.[44] Associations are made more quickly; the images which are evoked often seem to flash by and are reminiscent of the rapid associative images of video clips and film advertisements (which have in a sense been produced by them like fruits of the cocaine culture). However, the free – peaceful inner – capacity for clear thought and judgement, in which thoughts develop and are observed and "weighed up" on the basis of the free will, is obviously not helped by the effect of cocaine; this can only take place on the basis of free thoughts of the Self.

When cocaine is sniffed the euphoria, which lasts for about one hour (peaking after 15–20 minutes), is considerably milder than when cocaine is injected or smoked by freebasing. In both these cases the euphoria is much quicker, more short lived (lasting a maximum of 5 minutes) and intense. William Burroughs wrote: "It is the most cheerful drug I have ever used ... The total cheerfulness of cocaine can only be achieved by injecting it into a vein",[45] and nowadays, to a greater extent, by smoking crack. The orgiastic, foaming, intense feeling of bliss seems to result from the lightning process of "breathing in" of the astral body. This powerful and extremely rapid process of the astral body (rapid increase of blood pressure and heartbeat, often accompanied by pain in the heart area) is comparable to awakening in a flash: the astral forces which "flash" into the physical and ethereal body give the user the wonderful feeling of rushing energy and brilliant intellectual powers. She feels overflowing with energy, self-confidence, strength and power. In this respect, the cocaine (as well as the amphetamine) flash has a very different quality from the warm, floating sensation described for opium injections,[46] when the astral body moves *out*wards extremely quickly.

Thus cocaine gives feelings of power; the user feels sure of herself because of the surfeit of astral forces. She has no doubts, turns to the outside world and feels powerful and superior at parties, business meetings and so on. It is the macho drug par excellence. The ego is "blown up" and thunders over all the more delicate and subtle feelings. Gone are all the spiritual, artistic feelings of empathy. *No nonsense*! That's cocaine!

In this sense the drug is extremely attractive to anyone who wishes to overcome her own insecurity, fears and sense of inferiority, and that is why it is extremely popular with adolescents.

However, the inner price is high: the euphoria of the false sense of security is at the expense of a true feeling of security, at the expense of purely human experiences of insecurity, doubt and inner questions (which make development possible). These feelings and inner questions are overwhelmed by the hard and essentially rather cynical feeling produced by cocaine. The drug makes it impossible to have true sympathetic, empathetic or artistic feelings. Cocaine burns up the user and all her strength. The organic foundation of human emotions – the rhythmic system of respiration and circulation – is overburdened, and what remains in the end is exhaustion and emptiness. The heart, the organ of balanced judgement and warm, human involvement and love, is exhausted and ultimately the user discovers this in sombre, dark feelings of sadness, depletion and emptiness.

The hangover

The user feels tired and depressed, particularly after injecting cocaine or after smoking crack (and to a slightly lesser extent after sniffing cocaine). With regard to sniffing cocaine, Jürgen vom Scheidt wrote: "The peak of the exaltation which is directed at the outside world is followed after about an hour by a violent hangover. The user is exhausted, melancholic, and feels sleepy as though in a depression. This depressed mood sometimes even leads to suicide. However, in most cases the user will seek escape in another high."[47] With regard to freebasing or smoking crack, Bernard Segal wrote: "A single deep inhalation of the freebased smoke causes a strong rapid assimilation of the concentration of cocaine in the blood and in the brain. However, the problem is that the feeling of euphoria is very short-lived and that a feeling of depression may soon take over from the pleasant feelings. This depression contrasts so painfully with the high that the user will often try to repeat the euphoria by taking more of the drug. He will inhale every three to five minutes for long sessions which can last up to three days until the supplies of cocaine run out or the smoker collapses from exhaustion."[48]

Addiction

This can result in addiction.[49]

If the user regularly takes cocaine for a long time, four clear stages of intoxication can be distinguished:[50]

1. The stage of euphoria. Often this is accompanied by a sense of insecurity. The user is very alert, active, restless and talkative, and does not feel any tiredness. She comes across as a nervous, chattering hyperactive sort of bird jumping from one thing to the next.

2. The stage of dysphoria. The user loses the light, bright, boiling energy and becomes increasingly depressed, moody, fearful and irritable. These feelings alternate with periods of indifference and apathy. She finds it difficult to concentrate and starts to talk in a disjointed way.

3. The stage of suspicion. The user is troubled by hallucinations, particularly tactile hallucinations and paranoid fears. She feels insects or snakes crawling over her body (as Dr. Fleischl reported to Freud), or hallucinates about parasites and other creepy-crawlies moving under her skin. She may be troubled by itchy

arms, legs and back, and later feels this itching moving over her body.

4. The stage of psychosis, characterized by fearful paranoid delusions. These may be delusions about parasites, but may also take the form of a persecution complex. They are often accompanied by visual and aural hallucinations and even hallucinations of smell. The visual hallucinations, combined with a persecution complex, can be particularly strong.

Here is an example: "The patient is a young man of 25, who was admitted to the crisis centre because he was fleeing from the police. He constantly felt persecuted and saw policemen hiding everywhere. In his home he could hear them in the rooms of the people living above him and he could even see them spying on him through holes in the ceiling. He was very fearful because he actually saw their faces at night ...

When he was admitted, we saw a restless, fearful man who crawled over the floor of the examination room so that the police wouldn't see him. He suffered from vivid visual hallucinations (policemen, camouflaged police vans, spies walking past), and aural hallucinations (police sirens, car engines). He did not have any tactile hallucinations or delusions about parasites. His thoughts were characterized by serious paranoia and the sense that he was constantly being persecuted."[51]

These hallucinations are caused by the ethereal forces separating away from the physical organs of the body and penetrating the astral body, where they form images. In this sense insects, snakes, parasites and so on can be seen as animal (astral) images of the ethereal forces separating away from certain parts of the physical body (for example, snakes as an image for the veins and arteries, insects and parasites as an image for nerve cells etc.). The visual and aural hallucinations, such as the frightening policemen and police sirens in the example given above, can be viewed as the ethereal forces projected as an image in the astral body where they derive their terrifying character from the fact that the *heart*, the organ of the Self, is threatened by the effect of cocaine. It is essentially the heart that is depleted by cocaine, the Self is threatened and the user is terrified of being taken, getting lost, losing the Self.

Another hallucination which can occur at later stages of the psychosis is the vision of snow or cocaine crystals (snow lights), twinkling in the light. Sometimes, the user sees sparkling, glistening geometric patterns pulsating or vibrating with a very rapid frequency.[52]

These hallucinations appear to be images of ethereal form (ethereal crystallization) which has been released, or the forces of ethereal life "which create a geometric order in matter, in rhythmic crystal patterns" (Lievegoed, see p. 00). Finally, there are two phenomena which may occur during a cocaine psychosis:

a. The obsessive repetition of certain senseless stereotype acts such as constantly driving around the same block in a car.

The user may also become obsessed with particular futile efforts.

These obsessive acts can be viewed as the result of the ethereal forces released from the lungs. Rudolf Treichler wrote: "More than any other organ, the lungs, which are related to the pole formed by the head, have a tendency to become hard, calcified, ossified and sclerotic. This shows that the lungs are a central organ for the fundamental strength of the ethereal body, which creates and destroys the physical body in solid matter (ethereal life).

In this context, it is understandable that Rudolf Steiner points out that when such forces collecting in the lungs separate from the physical body, it leads to the formation of obsessive images."[53]

b. The paranoia, which may be combined with some of the above-mentioned hallucinations can lead to suicide or violent outbursts of aggression to the outside world. When this happens, the organ involved is the heart. Recklessness is one of the symptoms of heart psychosis.[54] Victor Bott wrote: "What started as the will became an obsession. This lack of control, this lack of inhibition, is the danger to which one is exposed. Sometimes it leads to self-destruction, which can also lead to the downfall of others. It is an all-consuming fire."[54]

Thus we see that in the cocaine psychosis the *heart* and the *lungs* are the damaged organs from which metabolic forces (ethereal forces) break away.[55] As a result, long-term use often means that the restless, excited, fearful and obsessive state which is caused, must be calmed and suppressed as far as possible. That is why many cocaine addicts often turn to alcohol, sleeping pills, tranquillizers and heroin after a while.

Finally, when the cocaine has finished working, a lengthy depression remains which can only be removed in the short term by taking more cocaine or other drugs. In this case, the user is suffering from a physically induced depression. Van Epen wrote: "The cocaine depression can resemble a vital endogenous depression accompanied by a sombre fearful mood, the lack of any perspective on life, complete indifference and apathy. The victims are extremely tired and lacking in energy. They do not sleep, they do not eat, they cannot cry and are often suicidal.[56]

The physical consequences of chronic use of cocaine

The major organs of the rhythmic system suffer particularly from the regular use of cocaine or crack.

With regard to the heart and circulation, there is an increased risk of heart attacks, strokes, and kidney failure (particularly with freebasing or smoking crack). A. Sahini wrote: "Because of the sudden contraction of the blood vessels the supply of blood to the heart is interrupted. The rapid rise in blood pressure and heartbeat can lead to cramps and cardiac arrest. Crack suppresses the production of several enzymes in the human body which are essential for the heart to function. As a result, the heart is under the greatest threat ..."[57]

However, the lungs are also damaged by inhaling the crack or freebased smoke. A. Sahini wrote: "On the bottom of a crack pipe which has been smoked two or three times there is a deposit of small, sticky lumps. The filter which forms the bottom of the bowl of the pipe must be regularly burnt out and frequently replaced or it will become clogged up. The black sticky lumps are also deposited in the bronchi but the lungs cannot be cleaned like a pipe. As a result, the user becomes short of breath and suffers from pain in his lungs when he makes the slightest effort. He becomes increasingly vulnerable to all sorts of lung complaints. On balance, someone who smokes crack becomes more sensitive to heart and lung disorders every time he uses the drug."[57]

Finally, the septum can be eroded by sniffing cocaine: it starts to blister and then perforates, which means that there is a hole in it.

As regards the metabolic organism, there is a reduction in the production of very important enzymes in the liver,[58] and occasionally also reduced kidney functioning.[59] Certain metabolic processes in the brain may also be interrupted for a time.[60] Furthermore, there may be an extreme loss of weight, as well as atrophying of the muscles.

Cocaine has a harmful influence on the reproductive processes of human beings. There is considerable increase in the chance of a miscarriage (38%),[58] and the babies who are born have more lung and kidney defects than babies of parents who do not use cocaine.[58] A study of 1,226 pregnant women who used drugs showed that the babies of women who had used cocaine weighed 93 grammes less at birth, and were 0.7 cm shorter than babies of mothers who had not used drugs.[61]

These dangers appear to be even greater as a result of smoking crack. A. Sahini wrote: "Stillbirths, miscarriages and paralysed or deformed babies were no exception amongst mothers who had smoked crack during pregnancy. Chromosome abnormalities, abnormal development of the sexual organs, weak heart and brain damage were most common. The babies ... had a weak immune system. The mortality rate was very high."[62]

Although there has been little large-scale research into the (long-term) consequences for the development of babies of mothers who use cocaine or crack, the first impressions give rise to great concern. An American doctor quoted by B. Segal in his book, *Drugs and Behaviour*, wrote: "The long-term consequences will be devastating. I see children who are clearly retarded in their mental development, who have great learning difficulties and all sorts of motor problems, even with regard to performing simple acts such as eating and getting dressed."[63]

In this respect, cocaine, which was originally considered rather harmless, appears to be a "white destroyer" after all, not only for the user, but also – to a greater or lesser extent – for the children of mothers who were chronic users of the drug during pregnancy. At any rate, it can already be concluded that women should be discouraged from using cocaine during pregnancy.[61]

Amphetamines (Speed)

Amphetamines also known as speed or pep, are stimulants with an effect that is very similar to that of cocaine.

For example, Louis S. Goodman and Alfred Gilman wrote in their *Pharmacological Basis of Therapeutics*, which is sometimes considered the "bible of medicines" "Cocaine addicts describe the euphoria of cocaine in a way which can hardly be distinguished from the descriptions of amphetamine addicts. In depressive patients cocaine produces a sense of increased pleasure, and the toxic syndrome caused by cocaine does not appear to differ clinically from that caused by amphetamines. Under test conditions, animals also present comparable patterns of behaviour when they are able to help themselves to cocaine and amphetamines. These substances lead to very similar subjective experiences, evoke similar toxic phenomena and in the case of non-medical use when one of the two substances is not available, they can be interchanged."[64] However, amphetamines do have the advantage that they last longer than cocaine (approximately four to eight hours when they are taken as tablets) and that they are also considerably cheaper.

The history

Amphetamines (also known as benzedrine) was synthesized in 1887 by the chemist Edeleanu. In 1910, the English physiologists, Barger and Dale, discovered that the chemical structure of benzedrine was closely related to the hormone adrenalin, which is formed in the adrenal glands and which increases blood pressure and the rate of the heartbeat amongst other things, so that the organism is in a heightened state of alertness. However, attempts to use amphetamines as a surrogate for adrenaline failed because the effect on the organs (heart, circulation, lungs) was too slight in animal tests, at least compared to adrenalin.

However, the stimulating properties of the drug were discovered later when amphetamines were given to animals which were subsequently anaesthetized; the anaesthesia lasted much shorter than usual. This meant that during the 1930s (a low dose of) this substance was used to combat a particular form of sleeping sickness in people which caused patients to suddenly fall asleep many times a day although there was no question of fatigue (narcolepsy).

When the stronger methamphetamine (methedrine, pervitine) was synthesized in 1919, this was followed by a great deal of research in the 1930s into the other properties and applications of amphetamines. It was discovered that short-lived physical performances were hardly improved by the influence of these drugs, though they were able to banish fatigue, sleepiness and feelings of exhaustion. This means that there was an increase in physical performance lasting a long time, resulting in the practice of doping in sport.

In addition, it became clear that amphetamines were very useful as a slimming remedy (it is as though the user burns with energy and has no appetite for a long time), but the risks and side effects were very great. Van Epen wrote: "It often results in a nervous, wound-up patient who loses kilos in weight but suffers from sleeplessness, sometimes develops high blood pressure and often puts weight back on after ceasing the medication. In addition, there is a risk of serious depression. When the patient discovers that a few of these slimming tablets will soon help him get over the depression, the vicious circle is complete and the basis of addiction has been laid."[65]

At the same time, it was discovered that low doses of amphetamines could be used as medication for the treatment of hyperactive children[66] who actually calmed down and became more adaptable as a result of these substances.

The first warnings appeared towards the end of the 1930s: "Amphetamines and related substances act as a whip on an exhausted horse. The result is that the physical reserves are depleted leading to collapse. Feelings of exhaustion which help to create a balance between the body and soul are violently suppressed. Amphetamines can lead to addiction."[67]

In America, a wave of addiction gradually developed as a result of "benzedrine inhalers" which were used from 1927 to treat colds. Later they were withdrawn from the market.

During the Second World War, pep pills were used on a large scale by soldiers on both sides to combat exhaustion, increase their stamina and encourage them to behave in a reckless, aggressive way. As described in Chapter 2, the American and English alone used an estimated 150 million pep pills ("combat pills").

After the Second World War there was a wave of addiction in Japan when millions of amphetamines came onto the market from army dumps: in 1950, it was estimated that there were between half a million and a million regular users. Strict laws were passed and there were huge numbers of arrests, but this did not prevent the use of amphetamines in Japan from continuing up to the present day.

In Sweden, there was a great increase in the use of speed in 1958, and intravenous injections became particularly popular. This led to a wave of speed in the 1960s, which was followed by a complete prohibition on production, trade and consumption. However, this prohibition also failed to deal with the popularity of amphetamines in Sweden. In the other Scandinavian countries they were (and are) also used illegally as a stimulant.

In the Netherlands there was a wave of speed from 1969 to 1972 (when heroin took over). During this period, violence on the part of the "speed freaks" was very common. Van Epen wrote: "The age of speed was especially difficult and unpleasant for people who worked with drug addicts: the users were generally excited, screwed up and aggressive. Many were temporarily, and sometimes for longer periods, psychotic (confused, with delusions and hallucinations). The physical condition of these addicts was a cause of great concern:

speed eventually exhausts the body and can cause all sorts of serious medical complications. During the age of speed many people who tried to help were attacked and sometimes injured by excitable "speed freaks." Knives and firearms also appeared on the scene. This was all a great contrast with the flower power period which preceded the age of speed." (68)

In 1976 amphetamines were included under the Opium Act and henceforth they were viewed in the same light as drugs such as LSD, mescaline, opiates, cocaine and so on.

The speed epidemic also cut across the ideals of the hippy era in America. In 1970 Timothy Leary warned: "Every time you take a toxic substance you are attacking nature. When you introduce amphetamines or barbiturates (sleeping pills or tranquillizers) into your organism, you are as bad as the oil producers who dump their poison into the oceans. Your body can move beautifully in harmony with nature: the blood flows and metabolic processes take place when you eat; all this happens in harmony with cosmic energy. However, when you introduce something into your body which demonstrably counteracts this harmony you turn off, not on. Amphetamines ... lead you along the wrong track on the path to the source of energy. Temporarily you become a superman and no one can stop you... Speed freaks believe that they have fantastic power and great creative potential, but in reality they never finish anything they have started. This is because speed is an unreal source of energy for them ... Speed never takes you to heaven, it sends you straight to hell. After all, the truly important thing is that we should all slow down."[69]

Sidney Cohen described the atmosphere of that time as follows: "The 'speed freak' is a chapter in himself. The 'true hippy' is astonished by the former's excessive consumption of amphetamines and criticizes these users for their need for stimulants. In the hippy ghettos, such as 'Haight Asbury' in San Francisco or Venice West in Los Angeles, you often see posters with captions like 'Speed Kills' or 'Meth (methedrine) is Death.' This is fairly clear proof that loyal LSD consumers see the abuse of amphetamines as dangerous and irreconcilable with the use of LSD. In these drug colonies methadrine consumers are viewed with suspicion, not only because of the paranoia they reveal, but also because of their impulsive and aggressive manner.

" ... One of the most common types of amphetamine abuse is

known as the 'tour', when the drug is injected every two to six hours without interruption until the user is exhausted and collapses, or until he takes barbiturates in order to go to sleep. These 'speed tours' often last for three to ten days; during this period the 'meth head' often does not eat or sleep, as his need to do so is cancelled out by the pharmacological effect of the drug. When he finally does fall asleep, this can often last from two to four or five days. When he wakes up, he feels enormously hungry and after satisfying his hunger he falls into a period of deep psychological depression. This depression is so overwhelming that he immediately seeks the only remedy; methedrine. In my view, depression, apathy and the decline of psychomotor activities are so extreme and regular in this case that it is a very specific withdrawal symptom."[70]

As a result of the growing number of bad experiences which speed freaks eventually go through because of their intensive use of the drug, and as a result of the increasing controls on the illegal production, trade, sale and consumption of amphetamines, the interest in this drug visibly diminished, paving the way for the new stimulant: cocaine. Admittedly, cocaine was more expensive, and the euphoria it produced did not last as long, but it had the advantage that it was made from natural raw materials and therefore seemed a much less harmful drug than the purely synthetic amphetamines. After all, the Indians had been chewing coca for centuries without being destroyed by it. The illegal drug trade was well-prepared for the growing demand and responded quickly and efficiently. Within a few years cocaine had taken the place of speed as the most widely used hard stimulant. However, amphetamines have not been banished altogether; they are still in circulation and are used illegally to combat exhaustion, to increase stamina in physical performance, to speed up thought processes (associations) and for the euphoria produced by the kick.

The effect

As mentioned above, the effect of amphetamines is very similar to that of cocaine. However, there is one big difference: amphetamines do not have any anaesthetizing properties.

As regards its stimulating properties, we see that the effect of speed also causes the astral body to become more strongly connected to the ethereal and physical body, resulting in increased activity and alertness. The user no longer feels exhaustion, which means that the astral body does not have the opportunity to separate from the ethereal and physical bodies in sleep so that it can, on the one hand, be dissolved in the cosmic astral world, and on the other hand, form another, regenerating, connection with the ethereal and physical body. (See the chapter on marijuana/hashish.) The astral body remains firmly connected to the physical and ethereal body (increased blood pressure and heartbeat, stimulation of certain parts of the brain, increased intestinal movements, and so on; see cocaine). Like cocaine it presses out the ethereal body with the result that vitality is increased but when the drug wears off – particularly in the case of successive doses – the user is left with a feeling of exhaustion and total emptiness. The ethereal forces have been burnt up and are completely exhausted. A long period of sleep is then required to restore as far as possible the vitality that has been lost.

In *The Science of the Secrets of the Soul*, Rudolf Steiner points out the importance for health of the rhythmic separation of the astral body in sleep, i.e. for the strengthening of the physical and ethereal body and for its well-being. He wrote: "The form and figure which belong to the physical human body can only be maintained by the ethereal human body, but this human form of the physical body can only be maintained by an ethereal body which is in turn supplied with the corresponding forces from the astral body. The ethereal body is the sculptor, the architect of the physical body. It can only develop in the right way if it is stimulated by the astral body to function as it should. There are examples in the latter, and the ethereal body copies these in the physical body. When a person is awake the astral body is not filled with these examples for the physical body, or only to a limited extent, for while it is awake the soul replaces the examples with its own images. When man directs his senses at the environment, his perceptions create images in his imagination and these are the copies of the world around him. These copies initially disrupt the images which encourage the ethereal body to maintain the physical body.

... Just as the physical body is based, as it were, in the physical world where it belongs, the astral body also belongs in its own world.

(.. And) just as the physical body obtains nourishment from its environment, the astral body acquires *images* from the surrounding world while the subject is asleep. It lives outside the physical body and the ethereal body, in the cosmos, the same cosmos from which man as a whole was born. The source of the images which give man his form lies in this cosmos. He is tuned into this cosmos in a harmonious way. When he is awake, he breaks away from this all-encompassing harmony to achieve external perceptions. When he is asleep, his astral body returns to this harmony of the cosmos. There is so much strength from the cosmos for the bodies when he awakes that it is possible to do without the harmony for a while. In sleep the astral body returns to the land of its birth, and when it wakes up it brings renewed strength into life. This strength, which the astral body provides on awakening is shown in the refreshing quality of healthy sleep."[71] This quotation was taken from Rudolf Steiner's work.[72]

When someone uses speed, we see that the astral body does not have the opportunity to withdraw from the physical and ethereal bodies when the person is exhausted. This means that the ethereal body cannot obtain the necessary strength from the astral body to build up and strengthen the physical body. As a result, the physical body deteriorates fairly quickly if the drug is used regularly and in high doses. The processes of degeneration caused by the lack of sleep and by the toxic effect of amphetamines can no longer be restored by the strengthening processes from the ethereal body.

The breaking down processes are stronger than the building up processes, the body degenerates faster that it can be restored, and the process of dying has been put into motion. Van Ree and Esseveld wrote: "There are sores which do not heal, considerable weight loss, crumbly finger nails, tooth decay and chronic lung infections."[73] In addition, there are all sorts of complications for the heart and vascular system, partly caused by the oppressive and incessant presence of the astral body. These complications can eventually lead to strokes, over-stimulation and breakdown of the nervous system (including skin irritations, so that speed addicts have a tendency to pick at their skin) and defects of the metabolic reproductive and locomotive organism (tremors in the hands and arms, problems of balance and, in men sometimes, extremely painful inflammations of the epididymis and the seminal tube).[74] All in all, the physical body breaks down.

Even when the doses are lower and the use of the drug is not so regular, these complaints occur in the form of unpleasant symptoms which accompany the uninterrupted presence of the astral body: irritability, restlessness, a sense of urgency, headaches, palpitations, fear, insomnia, stomach cramps, diarrhoea.[75] The toxic effect of amphetamines leads to dizziness, nausea and vomiting. In addition, there are the negative psychological effects described for cocaine viously strongest in the case of high and frequent doses. ...clude dysphoria (bad moods, irritability, fear and so on), sus-.icion, hallucinations (especially regarding the skin), depressions, psychosis, etc.

These symptoms are less strong when lower doses are taken but, in view of the fact that tolerance quickly develops in relation to the euphoric properties of speed (so that increasingly high doses are needed to obtain the desired effect), the negative symptoms become increasingly evident with repeated use – particularly in the case of addiction.

What does the euphoria consist of? The user feels energetic and wide awake, with a desire to converse and interact with others. Boredom, fatigue and feelings of depression disappear while physical and intellectual performances seems to improve. There is an extraordinary clarity in associative thinking: the associations – as well as the processes – seem to take place much faster than usual, which explains the name "speed." These are the pleasant feelings caused by the strong presence of the astral body, feelings of being wide-awake, active, with more self-confidence, less self-criticism, more daring, more aggression, more power. As stated above, this resembles the effect of cocaine, and yet many people who use the drug experience the effect of speed as something "synthetic", more acute and colder than that of cocaine.

However, it is certainly not the case that intellectual performance really does increase under the influence of speed. In this context, Wolfgang Schmidbauer quotes the autobiographical account of the German psychiatrist, Kurt Schneider, in the *Handbuch der Rauschdrogen* (Handbook of Hallucinogenic Drugs): "While under the influence of pervitine, I wrote at length and in detail but the next day I had to scrap most of it. My thought processes had been considerably reduced and were no longer strictly logical. On two evenings I managed to form unfounded hypotheses which did not stand up to criticism the next day. There had been an increase in initiative and a basic optimistic note in my feelings. A letter I wrote to a good friend received the answer: 'I enjoyed your childish optimism'."[76]

Students who take speed to prepare for exams and during their examinations are often disappointed. Wolfgang Schmidbauer wrote: "Admittedly it is sometimes possible to spend more hours learning because sleepiness is suppressed, but this success is often merely subjective. Because of the euphoria the student often believes that he has a better grasp of the material than he really has. During the examination he believes that he is giving quick correct answers while he is under the influence of amphetamines, while the examiner has a much less positive impression and may even give the student a bad mark because of his superficial comments."[76]

When a user increases the dose because she has developed a tolerance, the sense of clarity in the thoughts is often replaced by much more confused and chaotic associations.

However, the strongest euphoria is experienced in a "flash". This happens when speed is injected intravenously, resulting in an orgiastic feeling of energy, strength and power.

Finally, we will examine some of the symptoms which occur as a result of the regular use of speed:

a. First of all there is the hangover, accompanied by enormous exhaustion, lethargy, and depression (see cocaine). Another dose can alleviate these feelings but this can lead to addiction.

b. As a result, the paranoid and schizophrenic psychoses described for cocaine can follow after long-term intensive use. The heart and arteries in particular are damaged: an aggressive heart psychosis often manifests itself.

c. In addition to the obsessive repetition (see p.219) described for cocaine), there may also be so-called jerking or involuntary movements, e.g. chewing movements and grinding of the teeth, facial tics, rotating movements of the abdomen, nodding or shaking of the arms and hands. These all appear as hypernervous ticks caused by an excessive astral over-stimulation and the absence of the Self in these parts of the body. The Self has lost control and no longer sufficiently permeates these parts of the body; the organization of the Self breaks down.[77]

d. During the speed kick the role of the Self is virtually cancelled out. The other parts of the soul are influenced by the drug in the way described above, outside the Self. This means that the Self becomes, to a greater or lesser extent, non-active; it is a passive onlooker. There is virtually no development or growth of the Self.

e. Low doses of speed can be used to treat hyperactive children as described above. These children cannot stop moving and are easily distracted, which means that their astral body flits about and shoots off when they react quickly and sensitively to stimulae, but they can calm down as the result of amphetamines. Their astral body is brought to rest and no longer shoots away; speed makes the astral body move in the opposite direction so that it connects and concentrates with the result that the children calm down and become better adapted. However, there is a negative aspect to do with the artificial character and toxic effect of amphetamines. Moreover, it has been shown that children treated with speed in this way are more at risk of becoming addicted to amphetamines in adolescence.[78]

9

Ecstasy (XTC)

Ecstasy is a relative latecomer on the drug scene. It was first synthesized in 1898, but it was not until the first half of the 1980s that the drug became available on a large scale in the United States and subsequently appeared in the Netherlands. The new drug soon became popular and was used at parties, "house parties", at home and outdoors. This stimulant, which produces a "warm" social feeling, was consumed – and is consumed – almost exclusively in company, with groups of friends who have generally known each other for some time. The groups and movements which use Ecstasy very enormously – from New Agers to disco-goers, from so-called "fringe" elements to yuppies.

History

As stated above, XTC was first synthesized in 1898, although it did not yet have this name. This was in the laboratory of the pharmaceutical manufacturer, E. Merck, in Darmstadt (Germany), a company which also produced high quality morphine and cocaine, amongst other things. In 1912 the manufacturers applied for a patent for this new substance, which was produced on the basis of nutmeg oil, and this was granted in 1914.

It has long been known that nutmeg, which originates from the Molluca Islands, has medicinal as well as consciousness-changing qualities. In *Ecstasy, de opkomst van een bewustzijnsveranderend middel* (Ecstasy, the Development of a Consciousness-Changing Substance), Arno Adelaars wrote: "In the *Ayurveda*, a classical Indian book, nutmeg is described as a narcotic fruit. Slaves on Dutch ships which transported nutmeg in the 17th century were familiar with the hallucinogenic effects. They stole the nutmegs to escape from their appalling conditions for a while. They accepted the nausea and dizziness which accompanied the intoxication.

In 1829, the Czech biologist, Purkinje, was the first Western scientist to describe the hallucinogenic effect of nutmeg. He ate three nutmegs and thought that the state induced was strikingly similar to that caused by marijuana. One hundred and fifty years later his description was supported by the American black activist, Malcolm X. While he was in prison he used nutmeg, and said that it "Gave a kick like three or four pure marijuana joints."[1]

However, the new substance did not become very popular. There was an attempt to market it as an appetite suppressant (slimming remedy) but this did not happen when it became clear that there was no commercial interest. In the late 1930s the American firm, Smith, Kline and French, decided to market the substance after all, though the resulting undesirable side-effects ultimately stopped the firm from going ahead. In this way Ecstasy disappeared from sight.

However, it re-emerged when the American army ordered the University of Michigan to study the substance in 1953–54, at the time of the Cold War, in order to see if it could be used as a truth drug. However, it proved unsuitable for this purpose, though it did acquire the chemical name which it has kept to this very day: MDMA (3.4 Methylenedioxymethylamphetamine).

In 1960, the Polish chemists, S. Biniecki and E. Krajewski, improved the MDMA formula which was still based on nutmeg (safrol) oil.[2] However, a new production method was discovered. In the early 1960s the American researcher, Alexander Shulgin, from the chemical concern the Dow Chemical Company, managed to succeed in preparing MDMA synthetically on the basis of the chemical substance, piperonal.

In the early 1970s the possible applications of MDMA were virtually exclusively reserved for psychotherapeutic sessions in order to help patients to come into contact with feelings which were inaccessible under normal conditions. In this sense MDMA succeeded the stronger hallucinogenic drug, MDA, which was prohibited in 1970 even for therapeutic uses. In its turn MDA had succeeded the even stronger drug LSD, which had already been prohibited. In scientific terms this resulted in a dilemma in psychotherapeutic and psychiatric circles:[3] On the one hand, the research results of the alleged therapeutic applications of MDMA seemed sufficiently important to be published, while on the other hand, there was a danger that it would be prohibited as soon as the publications appeared.

Nevertheless, Alexander Shulgin and David Nichols published a scientific article in 1978. They stated that the substance "caused a change in consciousness that could easily be influenced, with emotional and sensual peaks ... , the effect was comparable to that of marijuana, a low dose of MDA or of psilocybin mushrooms without the hallucinogenic component."[4]

The effects became perceptible on average about half an hour after the drug was taken; it peaked about thirty minutes to one hour later and did not last longer than a few hours. The physical symptoms of poisoning and the psychological side effects seemed negligible. At most there were some side effects which are well-known from stimulants: loss of appetite, dilated pupils and stiff jaw muscles.[3]

More research was carried out and several articles appeared in the literature by other scientists. These described the way in which MDMA reduced feelings of fear, promoted openness in the expression of feelings and led to a general sense of well-being.

There was increasing interest in the substance. During the second half of the 1970s a group of enterprising chemists decided to establish a secret laboratory for the manufacture of MDMA in Marin County in California.[5] They tried to find an exciting name for the new product; initially "Empathy" seemed to be the most popular choice because of its "warm", sensitive, social properties, but in the end they opted for the more exciting name: "Ecstasy" (also known as XTC or E). A description dating from that time,[6] referring to the author Herman Hesse stated: "Ecstasy, the Entheogen (freely translated: awakening the God in yourself) of the 21st century. It is the world of your own soul which you seek. It is only within yourself that the other reality which you long for exists. I can only give you what you give in yourself. The only gallery of images which I can show you is that of your own soul. I can give you only the possibility, the stimulus, the key. I can help you to make your own world visible. No more than that."

You certainly should not take it at parties and other busy occasions (!) because: "Ecstasy should be taken, certainly when it is the first time, in a comfortable environment, for example, at home, in the evening by candlelight or with the lights turned low with soft, pleasant music. Not acid or rock and roll, but calming soul music."[6]

However, this was soon to change. Ecstasy was at first a substance which – according to the advertisements – could serve to "open the chakras of the heart" and "to stimulate the intuitive right half of the brain". It was particularly popular with the followers of Bhagwan Shree Rajneesh and many New Age enthusiasts but a new group of users appeared in the course of the 1980s.

Students at the Southern Methodist University in Dallas (Texas) discovered that Ecstasy was a satisfactory substitute for alcohol, which was forbidden at the university. During parties and raves they used Ecstasy as a stimulant, which made them less inhibited and gave them a sense of social belonging, as well as enough energy to carry on partying and dancing all night. Parker wrote that at the night clubs in Dallas, Ecstasy was openly sold to students who could pay for their 20 dollar dose by credit card.[7]

The recreational use of the drug increased rapidly, partly because of the many articles in magazines such as *Newsweek*, *Time* and *Life*. The drug researcher, Ronald Siegel, estimated that the number of doses sold in the United States in 1976 was about 10,000, while by 1985 he estimated that this had risen to 360,000.[8]

What the therapists had been afraid of happened in the end: on 1 July 1985, Ecstasy became an illegal drug and acquired the same status as LSD and heroin, amongst other drugs. The reasons for the prohibitions were:[9]
- warnings by scientists of a development similar to that which happened with LSD twenty years before, when the original enthusiasm for the drug, which had been considered harmless, was replaced by doubts because of the high number of victims (fatal accidents and schizophrenic psychoses);
- the occurrence of the first Ecstasy deaths (although these victims had also appeared to have taken other drugs at the same time).
- the mushrooming consumption of the drug.

Ecstasy was included in the heaviest category of the law. This means that it was considered to be a substance that is so dangerous to public heath that it may not even be used for medical or therapeutic purposes, and that it cannot be used for scientific research on human subjects.[10] The penalties for violating the law are severe: for a dealer, a maximum of fifteen years imprisonment and a fine of 125,000 dollars, for anyone in possession of Ecstasy, a maximum of five years imprisonment. Other countries have quickly followed suit; the Netherlands was one of the last to prohibit the drug in 1988.

However, the prohibition in the United States by no means meant that the consumption actually decreased. Prices rose and the quality of the drug diminished (because it was cut, e.g. with amphetamines, ephedrine, MDA and caffeine) which in itself led to more than 500 hospital admissions of overdose symptoms in the first few months after the prohibition.

In fact, there was even an increase in consumption: in 1986 Siegel stated that clandestine laboratories had been established throughout the United States and that there were also large-scale preparations for massive distribution of the drug throughout Europe. A survey carried out on the campus of Stanford University in 1987 revealed that 40% of the students had used Ecstasy.[8]

Via the Bhagwan circuit, meditation centres and individuals, the drug has also been increasingly available in Europe since 1985. In these circles the consumption was aimed particularly at the acquisition of a greater insight into the Self; it was usually taken in a quiet environment. One Bhagwan follower wrote: "Just before this first pill, my mother gave me books by Osho (as the Bhagwan called himself just before his death) and these things merged. The Ecstasy experience fitted in beautifully with what happens in sanyassins, breaking down barriers, opening your Self. For me the summer of 1987 was the Magic Summer. My life seemed to take off, my relationships with people became deeper. My life took a different direction partly because of Ecstasy."[11]

However, there was also another path by which Ecstasy reached Europe, and that was via the dance floors. It proved to be an excellent means of supporting the atmosphere of purely electronic house parties where everyone dances together to the musical imagination of a disc jockey. This atmosphere could result in a trancelike state of consciousness.

In house music, which started in the Warehouse dance club in Chicago in the early 1980s, the disc jockey plays an extremely important role. He is the man who creates the music, adjusting the controls to the beat of a drum machine; his creativity determines the music which is based on a fixed beat. Arno Adelaars wrote: "As in the case of hip-hop, the disc jockey developed to become an experienced musician with the help of computers and turntables with commercial songs. The predominating feature of house music is the beat at 120–126 beats per minute. This beat whips up the dancer, and as there isn't a second break in the rhythm, the dancer falls into a trance. This technique has been used by African tribes for centuries."[12]

Eric Fromberg wrote about the history of house music: "In Chicago, the birthplace of house music, the starting rhythm, the beat of 120 beats per minute, is combined with a separate melody, and these two are constantly alternated. A record lasts approximately 6 minutes and there is little variation: occasionally something is removed or something is added, but the beat goes on. There is only one thing to concentrate on. This music, which is often made by black musicians and has clear characteristics of disco music, eventually spread to England where it became 'Acid House' music by combining the beat with the melodies of acid rock dating from the 1960s. Thus, 'acid' is only a small and specific stream in house music, which is already a thing of the past.

"One important aspect of house music was that it could all be manufactured in your own living room. All you needed was a drum machine and a small synthesizer. You record the results and then you can turn the recordings on and off yourself. Technically it is very easy to do. This revolution meant that making music became possible for the masses. Subsequently this style spread across Europe like wildfire but in several countries people incorporated their own influences: for example, they added or removed elements or placed different emphases. In this way house music was also combined with 'hip-hop' in which 'rap' is the dance style. However, despite all these different styles there is always one predominating element: the beat. The beat goes on all evening while the disc jockey changes the melodies ... house music sessions go on for hours."[13]

Meyer wrote: "You go out for a whole evening and at a party you may be dancing for six hours or so. You become a sort of musician because there is no structure in the music, but by using different elements from records you can tell a story in the course of an evening. You can let the evening collapse or you can pep it up. It could be compared to an African tribe on TV where there people are playing the drum and a whole tribe can dance to this for hours like crazy. To some extent house music is comparable ..."

It was very exciting. When you went into the party there would be a huge dance floor. This is also different from the large regular discos. The largest surface area is devoted to dancing; the bar is not really very important. Everything else is subordinate – it is the dance floor that is important. Groups of people are dancing together and this is felt to be the main thing. They enter into a sort of group trance. You encourage each other, and people shout out certain things through the music. You start to feel that you are part of a crowd."[14]

As expected, the effect of Ecstasy and the atmosphere of the (acid) house parties went together perfectly. It was as though Ecstasy and the wild trance-induced dancing led by the disc jockey were made for each other. Ecstasy also influenced house music.

Arno Adelaars wrote: "In Chicago there was a sort of cross-pollination between acid house and Ecstasy. Some of the musicians took Ecstasy pills, and you could hear this in their music. The rhythm and blues influences disappeared, to be replaced by a full sound of jingles and heavy whispering.

In the Chicago club people who took Ecstasy danced to this music. This cult also became popular in the hippy paradise, Goa, and the trendy holiday island of Ibiza. This special effect of Ecstasy seemed perfect for dance marathons that went on for nights on end. The pill helped people to forget their inhibitions and made them feel more sociable. The stimulating effects of Ecstasy gave them enough energy to dance all night … .

The tourists who went to Ibiza mainly came to dance and for the parties and love. The island is one of the places in the world where heterosexuals and homosexuals go to the same places without any problems … A secretary from Utrecht who went to Ibiza for a few weeks every summer four years running described the atmosphere in 1986 as follows: "I was particularly attracted by all the freaks, bizarrely dressed gays and many transvestites. Everyone seemed crazy and this gave me a kick, a real kick. Because of all these crazy people there was a very exuberant atmosphere."

On Ibiza, Ecstasy appeared at the same time as house music. It was probably used as a party drug for the first time in Europe in the large open-air discotheques. The new generation of consumers wanted to have fun, and one of these pills seemed to guarantee a thrilling evening. This new way of using Ecstasy was eminently suitable for the psychedelic, electronic acid house dance music. The exuberant party crowd of holidaymakers, who wanted to throw off all their inhibitions for a few weeks so that they could face the rest of the year, was undoubtedly in the mood for experimentation. During this summer Ibiza was known as "E island".

The next summer more people were introduced to the music and the pill. That year the atmosphere on Ibiza was even wilder than the previous year. The public danced with even more exuberance and the music sounded even more ecstatic. The partying holidaymakers added something to the concept of acid house and Ecstasy as a party drug: an explosive holiday atmosphere, a feeling that you could do anything, a playful way of dancing and making contact with people. Everyone was nice to each other and everyone danced with everyone else.

Danny Rampling, a disc jockey from London, fell under the spell of this contagious way of going out. He introduced the music and the dance style in London with the name, "Balearic Beat". The nights which he organized in his Shoom Club were a huge success. He managed to evoke the Mediterranean atmosphere which had made the discos in Ibiza so special. With the abundant use of smoke machines and bizarre light effects, it looked as though the sun was setting in an apocalyptic cloud of smoke one minute, while the next minute no one could see a thing. The trendy public in London succumbed to this new style en masse."[15]

From Chicago, Ibiza and London, the new trend spread to the mainland; the first acid-house parties took place in Amsterdam in 1987. At the beginning of September 1988 the first really huge acid-house party was held in Amsterdam in a converted warehouse. The motto of this party was "Trance." The guest disc jockey was Danny Rampling. It was followed by many other parties. Arno Adelaars wrote about these parties: "One party I went to in the winter of 1988/89 took place in the Amsterdam VOC Theatre. It was really seething. The music was pounding with the average tempo of a heartbeat. Just like a heart, this music did not miss a beat all night. The hits followed each other like beads on a string, without any interruption which might break the trance. It looked as though three-quarters of the people there were under the influence of E."[16]

However, another type of Ecstasy consumption still exists today: taking the drug at home, in small intimate circles. The American drug researcher, Rosenbaum, gave a good example of this: "It consists of a group of highly educated men and women with busy responsible jobs (doctors, lawyers, project developers and other businessmen), who have hardly any time to keep up their old friendships because of their busy lives and many responsibilities. The solution which this group found was to rent a house in the country once or twice a year, take Ecstasy and catch up on talking. The drug intensifies their communication and makes it possible to express ideas directly, missing out the 'warming-up period' which old friends often need to re-establish contact when they have not seen each other for a long time."[17]

For both groups (both the home consumers and the partygoers), 1991 was a year in which regular users, i.e. people who take Ecstasy once or more a month, were estimated at about 10,000 people.[18]

The effect

The effect of Ecstasy can be described as a unique combination of the effects of marijuana/hashish and speed. There is the stimulating undercurrent of speed, and there is also the dominant effect on the emotions which marijuana/hashish has.

What happens during an Ecstasy high? We shall try to explain this with reference to the words of several users, as recorded in *Ecstasy, de opkomst van een bewustzijnsveranderend middel* (Ecstasy, The Introduction of a Consciousness-Changing Substance), by Arno Adelaars, and *XTC, hard drug of onschuldig genotmiddel?* (Ecstasy: Hard Drug or Harmless Stimulant?) and *XTC, een nieuwe soft drug* (XTC, a New Soft Drug), by Eric Fromberg.

When an Ecstasy pill is taken, a short period of disorientation follows after approximately 20-60 minutes: "You feel a slight tingling throughout your body. Sometimes you have a stiff feeling in your arms, legs and jaw and your mouth feels dry. Your pupils dilate and your heart beats faster. Sometimes you feel nauseous. In some cases you get a feeling of constriction when the drug starts to have an effect (fresh air can help). These physical effects are not particularly strong."[19]

In this context the possibly frightening feelings of disorientation and constriction, and particularly the stiffness in the arms, legs and jaw, i.e. in the user's movement, are interesting. These symptoms are reminiscent of the initiation process described for the effect of opiates, when man's spiritual aspect is driven out of the motor organism which has become rigid with fright as a result of a strong shock. As a result this spiritual aspect of man is perceived by the brain which has been changed by a physical substance (see Chapter 6, Opiates, footnote 55). The same process seems to take place to some extent with the effect of Ecstasy. It confirms its reputation as a sacred drug, for users who are more concerned with self-knowledge and intimate social contacts, and as a drug of "artificial enlightenment." The effects of a partial separation and expansion of the spiritual aspect are sometimes experienced at the same time, but usually afterwards, when the astral body, with the Self in its "lap", separates away. This can happen very quickly, in a rush, or in a flash: "Twenty minutes after taking the pill I started to float and flash. It was a jolt, bang, from being sober to being very stoned."[20] In addition: "I felt warm ... but very relaxed. A sort of resignation crawled all over me. I let go of control ... At this moment I wanted to touch someone. I wanted to fall away together. When this happens I fall into the arms of whoever is standing next to me, no matter who it is. A flash lasts five to ten minutes, sometimes even shorter."[21]

At the same time, the astral body also *enters* the physical body, in particular because of the amphetamine-like effect of Ecstasy: "My hands were clammy and I felt a sort of shiver through my arms. I wanted to move, but I had to stand and go outside. It was a restless feeling but not frightening, though you do think – oh dear, here it comes."[20] The heartbeat and blood pressure rise and the astral body spurs the physical body on to greater activity.

These two opposite movements, i.e. the expansion and possible partial separation, and the partial entry of the astral body, are combined when Ecstasy is taken and are experienced at the same time. This can also be described by saying that at the periphery, the astral body becomes partly elastic (and floppy) under the influence of Ecstasy, so that the Ecstasy user has to laugh and smile (the well-known Ecstasy smile is comparable to the giggling of the marijuana/hash user), while on the other hand, the astral body is to some extent forced to press against the physical and ethereal body, resulting in the stimulating effect of Ecstasy.

For the user these two simultaneous movements lead to the strange experience of being relaxed at the same time as wanting to make an effort, a feeling of letting go and being active all at once: "I felt warm and a great drive but very relaxed. I felt entirely resigned. I let go of control, but had the feeling of being under control. It sounds contradictory, but that's what it felt like."[21]

This rapid separation and entry is a good feeling, the start of a sense of euphoria. "It is a wave of blissful feeling as though you're exploding with happiness."[21]

During the rest of the intoxication, which is often experienced in waves, this double movement of the astral body continues to take place. On the one hand, there are the stimulating effects which were described in detail for amphetamines and cocaine (such as increased blood pressure, a higher pulse, dilated pupils, tension in the jaw, slight co-ordination problems, and the loss of appetite), while on the other hand, there are many effects which can also occur when marijuana/hashish are taken.

With regard to the latter, there are the following similarities:

a. Like cannabis, the astral body stretches out, partly separates away and expands in the astral world with the Self in its lap, and combines with the astral bodies and Selves of other users to whom the same applies. This gives the users a sense of intimacy, an intense empathy, sympathy and oneness.

Here are some experiences:
– "Usually there was a great deal of misunderstanding when we tried to talk to each other. For example, we used the same words in a different way, which led to confusion and quarrelling. However, with Ecstasy this did not happen at all. We understood each other fully."[22]
– "When you take E you can get into someone else's skin. You see things very clearly. You understand people very well and can really listen to them."[23]
– "We talked together for hours, all three completely engrossed in each other. Sometimes others joined us. One look at someone in the corner and you understood them completely. I talked through a past incident with Henk to put it right. Suddenly it was important because we had never talked about it."[24]

b. As we described for the effect of marijuana/hashish, the astral body partly connects with the nervous system of the spinal cord, while the Self, which has also separated, connects with the autonomous or vegetative nervous system, amongst other things.

Consequently, the intimate fusion of the astral bodies is accompanied by a feeling of mutual understanding and love (see Marijuana/hashish, p. 103). This is why Ecstasy produces a warm sense of love and being in love. It is also for this reason that it is described as a "cuddly" drug.
– "I felt their love for each other with a warm intensity I'd never felt before. They felt my interest and each took hold of one of my hands. 'You're so beautiful', said Ian. 'You're radiant from within.' 'Do you mean you can see this?' I asked. 'No, it's what I feel', he answered ... I didn't feel sexually excited at all. It was as if this was no longer necessary. It was as though my need for love was completely satisfied."[24]
– "There was a tremendous feeling of peace, you're at peace with the world. You feel open, clear and full of love. I can't image anyone being angry under the influence of Ecstasy, or selfish or mean or defensive."[25]
– "I first took Ecstasy on a summer's day in July 1981 together with twelve Sanyassins. It was a day I will never forget. I received a lot of heart space, a feeling of total freedom from within and all the barriers had disappeared. It was a tremendous feeling.

There were twelve of us sitting having a drink outside in Amsterdam, just being. There was a great deal of love in the group, there was no need to talk and it was often quiet. We were enjoying existing, simply being. We shared our feelings. I had never experienced anything like this. I could simply describe my first Ecstasy experience as "artificial enlightenment".[26]

c.   Thus it is the forces of sympathy, i.e. of the fusion and becoming one, which are evoked in abundance through the effect of Ecstasy. All antipathy dies away; the forces of distancing yourself, being alone, and critical feelings are experienced to a much lesser extent. You enjoy expanding into others. It is a "bright, relaxed, easy feeling" and you feel "mellow".

Here are some examples:
– "A clever person is reserved and distant. This behaviour certainly does not appear under the influence of Ecstasy. Everything is good fun, friendly and delightful."[24]
– "If someone always behaved like I do after taking Ecstasy, I think they would be completely uninteresting and empty-headed. A fool, who can be good fun in the pub, laughing and shouting and having a ball but when it comes to talking about things which are not so much fun, forget it. And after all, that is what makes us human."[27]
– "I make sure that my Ecstasy sessions are very well-planned. I won't do it with just anyone. Ecstasy is very positive. Everything is smoothed over and you see only the beautiful things. I don't want that. I don't want to like someone suddenly when I normally have nothing in common with them. It's artificial."[28]

d.   In addition, the many spiritual aspects which have become stuck and have descended can be drawn up from the depths of the astral body – with the movement of the peripheral astral body – and these can now be perceived by the Self (which is connected to the astral body) from the inside. The speed component accelerates this process.
– "When it started to work I talked non-stop, quite unbelievable, ecstatic. We recorded it on a tape but when I listen to it now I feel ashamed. I had felt so free. Everything I had hidden away, came forward. A lid came off the well, and everything which was underneath came out. The next day I was different, truly a different person."[29]
– "We often called Ecstasy the accelerator because everything came out more quickly with it. The substance strengthens what

is inside you. Sometimes everything is accelerated. During one session, Kees-Jan's brother and his girlfriend talked about their relationship. They were so open and honest that they both realized that they could not go on. Their relationship was finished in one session."[30]

e. The feeling of pain can also disappear. The astral body (consciousness) no longer perceives these stimuli: "I had a headache and felt foolish. A friend came by and told me that he had once taken Ecstasy when he was ill and it had helped. He convinced me, and I took half a tab. At first I sweated a lot, it seemed as though I was covered in foam, but my headache disappeared and didn't come back."[31]

In addition, when the state of intoxication is (almost) over and the user becomes tired, the astral body can sometimes withdraw fairly easily from the physical and ethereal body with the result that he falls asleep. However, in some people the opposite happens: because of the partial entry and the connection with the astral body and the ethereal body, this essential aspect finds it more difficult to separate away from the physical and the ethereal body, resulting in insomnia.

De Korf et al. wrote: "Sleeping badly towards the end of a state of intoxication is usually mentioned as a negative effect. However, there are people who sleep like a log, feeling tired and content."[32]

To summarize, it is clear that, like marijuana/hashish, Ecstasy strongly stimulates the user's emotions by affecting the astral body. Feelings of relaxation, openness, empathy, warmth, sympathy and love are powerfully evoked. The sensory experiences often become more sensual and emotive. There is a greater sensitivity to music, colours and smells. In other words, Ecstasy is an enhancer of feelings, reinforcing sensory perception and intensifying experiences. Things look more beautiful and things which are normal are suddenly fun."[33] However, there is more to it than this; the speed component can stimulate action. The feelings lead to a desire for action and company (to mingle with other astral bodies and selves), a desire to talk, observe and fuse in mutual sympathy. Or to dance: "I felt like a little rubber ball. I leapt amongst all the people with my arms up and just kept on smiling."[34]

Nevertheless, as in the case of marijuana/hashish there may also be consequences caused by the effect of Ecstasy on the links between the ethereal body and the physical body. Ecstasy is actually a toxin which can lead to the partial process of dying described under the effects of LSD, when a large but not fatal dose is taken. This means that the ethereal body partly separates away from the physical body. As a result there may be a few symptoms which will be familiar from the description of the effects of LSD (and to a lesser extent to that of cannabis), such as:

— Snippets of your past life:
  "It's a trip through your own consciousness, but through the eyes of another person. You are in the Here and Now of Then. You become a child but your adult brain can understand why people reacted to you as they did. You do not have hallucinations, but it is more as though slides of your life are projected in a jumble."[35]

— Hallucinations, disorientation:
  "When the double dose of Ecstasy started to work after half an hour, it was much stronger than it should have been. I was walking to a discotheque with two friends. I no longer recognized the street where I go almost every day to do my shopping. The pavement was made of rubber, cotton wool or perhaps even of wooden posts. I could hardly stand up. There were warm pink clouds in my head blocking my thoughts."[36]

  These hallucinations can be reinforced by the use of marijuana/hashish: "Nowadays, I always combine Ecstasy with grass. At a certain point I noticed that the effect was quicker when I smoked a joint half-an-hour after taking the Ecstasy. I think this is connected to the two-component theory: Ecstasy has a hallucinogenic and stimulating side. I like the hallucinogenic side and this is increased by smoking dope. A friend of mine prefers the stimulating side and he takes Ecstasy in combination with speed."[37]

Looking at the effect of Ecstasy on the user's Self reveals that during the state of intoxication the Self is forced to undergo these effects. It is forced to go along on the wings of the expanding astral body which becomes peripheral, and is forced to see the other part of the astral body becoming more strongly linked to the physical and ethereal body. It enjoys this, but like the astral body, the Self is in a sense pulled apart, losing its centre, stability and initiative. The consequences can last for a long time, particularly after repeated use:

— "After a while I had the feeling of losing my centre, I became too sensitive and had little resilience. I was regularly sick off work.

Not that I was really ill, but I thought I could no longer cope."[38]
- "Many people around me were using Ecstasy. A number of them seemed to undergo personality changes which frightened me. There was a contrast between their partying behaviour and their behaviour in daily life. They became indifferent and sometimes even asocial."[39]

In addition, when the organization of the essential aspects has become unstable because of the influence of Ecstasy and other drugs, the Self may lose contact with reality when Ecstasy is used regularly. In this case the Self flies off on the wings of the astral body as it flies to the periphery: "I seemed to live completely from the air. When I was high I often walked around the room flapping my arms like an angel. I floated about more and more. I became lighter and separated away from the earth. Even literally. My appetite decreased and I lost weight. In the end I ate hardly anything and only weighed about 50 kilos."[40]

However, above all, there is, of course, the dissolving and fusing of the astral body and Self with the astral bodies and selves of the other users: the individual, independent, separate, consciousness of the Self is more or less dissolved in a group consciousness which may be in a trance-like state as a result of house music. In this way an ancient state of consciousness is artificially evoked: the consciousness which was characterized in the description of alcohol and of marijuana/hashish as the all-pervasive, dreamy, ancient, group-consciousness of man rooted in the world of the gods. It becomes increasingly lost there, particularly in the case of regular use, taking a step backwards in its development. In addition the experiences of self-insight, openness, empathy, warmth, sympathy and love cannot become qualities or skills of the Self as they have not been acquired as the result of practice and effort. The Self has not acquired these qualities by trial and error. It merely had these experiences while the drug was working. After this it was finished leaving only a memory. However, the experiences described can have a great effect and even change the direction of someone's life, though they do not lead to lasting skills. They come and go with the effects of the drug.

Risks

One of the greatest problems in assessing the risks of Ecstasy, apart from what was described above, is the fact that there are no research data on the long-term effects. For example, there are no data about people who have been regularly been taking Ecstasy for twenty years or so (which is a big difference with alcohol and a number of other drugs). In addition, research into the effects of chemically pure Ecstasy is made more difficult in practice because it is an illegal substance with the result that it is only possible to study the effects of the street product on illegal users. However, this street product by no means always consists of pure Ecstasy. For example, during the period 1989 to January 1991, only 54% of the samples tested in Amsterdam consisted of pure Ecstasy.[41] Almost a quarter of these samples proved to contain amphetamine or MDA, while a similar proportion contained other substances such as aspirin, vitamin pills and mixtures of various substances.[42] Even when the street product did contain pure Ecstasy there were large differences in the doses: from 36 mg to more than the maximum dose of 50 mg (per pill).[43]

This uncertainty regarding the actual content of the Ecstasy pill can result in dangerous situations for users. A regular user took six pills in a few days and had the following experience:

"The Ecstasy slowly disappeared from my body. I was lying on my hotel bed and suddenly I lost it … Everything went white, and I was scared of falling out of bed, going into a coma or dying. It was terrible. Inside my skull there was a high-pitched noise and it seemed as though my ear drums were bursting. This lasted for a long time … I was incredibly frightened but it wasn't over yet. The next day a similar thing happened while I was in the street. Again everything was white and I heard the high-pitched noise in my head. I had to hold on to something it was so bad. When I was back in the Netherlands I talked to some friends and it seemed I was not alone in having these sorts of symptoms. I'm not sure exactly where it came from. I think there was a lot of pep in those pills. Perhaps that's why I used so many."[44]

In March 1992 the Amsterdam Drugs Advice Bureau and the Dutch Institute for Alcohol and Drugs issued the following warning (see opposite page).

The effects of a pure Ecstasy overdose, i.e. a very high but non-fatal dose of pure Ecstasy are very similar to those of an amphetamine dose: accelerated heartbeat, increased blood pressure, changing to a reduction in blood pressure after about six hours, hallucinations and paranoid panic attacks and rage. The heart and arteries are greatly burdened. Even with a normal dose, Ecstasy can cause sudden cardiac arrest in people with heart and circulation disorders. For the street product the physical effects of an overdose included:

WARNING
for all XTC users

As you know, many dangerous pills are sold as XTC. Analyses have shown that things have got really bad in the last few weeks.

We are finding pills with a high (!) dose of SPEED.

There are pills containing MDA, a hallucinogenic relation of XTC (MDMA), and pills with nothing in them, i.e. fake pills.

Please be specially careful about taking:

- A large LIGHT BLUE pill, which is speed;
- Look-alikes for the so-called SALMIAKS. This pill has also now become unreliable;
- And take extra special care with regard to a FLAT WHITE pill, 9 x 4 mm, with a groove on one side. This contains KETAMINE, a NARCOTIC substance.

Wherever you are, at home, or at a disco or party, you have been warned.
Apart from this, have fun.

Drugs Advice Bureau, Amsterdam

greatly accelerated heartbeat, greatly increased blood pressure, changing to a greatly reduced blood pressure, palpitations, increased muscular tension (stiffness in the arms, legs and jaw), severe perspiration, kidney failure, visual hallucinations, destruction of muscle cells.[45] Moreover, experiments on animals showed that frequent high doses of Ecstasy influence certain metabolic processes in the brain: In 1988, Ricaurte discovered that in monkeys Ecstasy inhibited the reassimilation of the neurotransmitter, serotonin, in the nerve ends of the brain cells, with the result that the amount of serotonin in the monkey's brains was reduced.[46]

An examination of the unpleasant effects during and after the state of intoxication in a study by D. Korf et al. on secondary school pupils (average age 16.5 years old), and on people in a coffee shop (average age 23.3 years old), produced the following results:[47]

- During the first few hours of the state of intoxication the negative experiences included nausea, sudden chills, shivering, stiff jaw, sweating, frequent urination and feelings of fear.
- This is followed after about four hours by increasing tiredness, fear and depression, and when the state of intoxication comes to an end these symptoms are supplemented by stiff limbs, chattering teeth, severe shivering, loss of concentration and above all feelings of emptiness and insomnia.
- Insofar as the effects of the Ecstasy are still perceptible when the period of intoxication comes to an end (after about seven to eight hours) they are predominantly experienced as negative effects;
- The day after, more than half of the users have a hangover while 33% of users feel mainly alright (especially in the company of others with whom the drug was taken the day before). In this case, there can be a sense of pleasant tiredness and lethargy, while others can feel light-headed. The symptoms of the hangover are comparable to those of cocaine and speed:
- palpitations, headache, stomach ache, muscular cramps, cramps in the eyes and jaw, slight disorientation, severe perspiration and a feeling of stress;
- mainly a sense of emptiness, listlessness and being tired out. A feeling of tiredness, dopiness and irritability.

To gain an impression of the long-term effects of the regular use of Ecstasy it seems likely that the desirable effects will decrease, while the undesirable effects will gradually increase and can even lead to strong negative symptoms after a while, such as loss of appetite, lack of energy, depression, involuntary flashbacks and delusions.[48] "If you use Ecstasy often, at short intervals, the effects change. There is no longer any sense of pleasure, and this is replaced with tension, irritabilty or insomnia."[19]

10

Designer Drugs

In general, designer drugs are (fairly) recent consciousness- changing substances which are designed almost "on the drawing board" in order to manipulate the consciousness of users in a variety of different ways. This is done by very slightly modifying the chemical formulae of certain substances (usually other consciousness-changing substances), for example by replacing an alpha-methyl group by a methyl group, etc. In this way it is possible to use combinations of legal substances to produce drugs which are not made illegal until later. It actually takes a long time before the government can test the new substances for the dangers they present, and before their harmful influence can be adequately proved. In the meantime these drugs can be distributed and a wide circle of clients can be built up; this circle usually continues to exist once the drugs have been prohibited because the new substances have become sufficiently popular on the drug scene (or a new variation of the prohibited substance – which is not yet prohibited – is introduced, so that history repeats itself). In addition, these designer drugs have the advantage for dealers that, in general, they can be manufactured fairly simply and cheaply and they usually lead rapidly to a physical and/or psychological dependency. As a result, a paying circle of addicted consumers can be built up within a short period. Because there are usually no long transportation routes or any borders to be crossed – by now every country and every area has its own clandestine laboratories – the transportation costs are extremely low, with the result that there are huge profits to be made for the dealers.

Another advantage of the designer drugs for the dealers is that even very small quantities produce an extremely strong effect on the user's body. For example, there are compounds of the designer drug, Fentanyl, which have an effect that is between 1,000 and 7,500 times as strong as morphine. It is therefore not necessary to manufacture much of the substance. For example, when one thimble full of a substance such as Fentanyl has been synthesized, it can be used for tens of thousands of doses. If these are not measured exactly, i.e. not in extremely minuscule quantities (and/or combined with poisonous substances) this can result in serious symptoms of poisoning or fatal accidents (so-called "unintentional" overdoses).

Many people see the drug wave of the 1990s in terms of designer drugs. In the United States these drugs of the future are already one of the greatest problems in the "war against drugs."

What are the most important designer drugs up to now?

a. In the category of synthetic opiates there are the Fentanyl compounds, i.e. the virtually infinite family of derivatives of the narcotic, Fentanyl. There are Fentanyl compounds which have effects that are respectively 10, 175, 200, 450, 600, 1000, 1,500, 3,000, and 7,500 times as strong as morphine. In these last drugs the separation of the astral body takes place so quickly that it leads to an unimaginably intense euphoria followed by deep unconsciousness. Thus, in fact, the user sleeps off the intoxication after the flash. In this context, an anaesthetist at Stanford University Hospital, Will Spiegelman, said: "It can take years before a person becomes addicted to alcohol, but it takes only a single shot of Fentanyl to become addicted."[1]

In addition, there are drugs like MPTP, a derivative of the pain killer Demerol (Meperidine). It is extremely toxic and has side-effects with the characteristics of Parkinson's disease. It quickly leads to physical dependency, and MPTP has been called the new heroin.

b. The designer drugs which seek to combine hallucinogenic and stimulating effects are popular. Examples of these are STP (DOM) and MDA (3.4 *Methylenedioxyamphetamine*) which conjures up inner images from the past (particularly when the eyes are shut), though the effect is less strong than that of LSD or mescaline. However, MDA also greatly strengthens the emotions and feelings of empathy, and is therefore a very popular recreational drug.

A small change in the chemical formula of MDA (replacing a hydrogen atom with a methyl group) results in MDMA or Ecstasy, and with this the hallucinogenic effects have (virtually) disappeared.

One very dangerous drug which particularly meets the death wish is PCP (Phencyclidine), also known as Angel Dust after the Californian bikers, the Hell's Angels, who introduced PCP on the drug scene in the early 1970s. PCP can take effect for between three-quarters of an hour and forty-eight hours and produces experiences of a horror trip amongst other things. It can work as a hallucinogenic, a stimulant or a narcotic drug, depending on the quantity taken, the way in which it is used and the consumer's nature. It is extremely poisonous and can lead to insanity; the essential aspects of a human being fall into complete chaos. Here are some examples: "Under the influence of the drug the student, Charlie Innes, gouged out both his eyes and gave them to the police officers who had arrested him on a charge of immoral conduct. Other PCP addicts jumped from the roofs of houses, chopped their legs off with axes and bled to death, drowned in puddles of water in the road or calmly lay down on the railway track to be run over". One addict described the effect as follows: "It is as though one is liberated from one's body"; other consumers of Angel Dust wrote about feelings of persecution and intense hallucinations, usually of a very frightening nature. During the trip other people often looked like monsters pulling horrendous faces, cars changed into dragons, trees into threatening giants – delusions which are like those of Hieronymus Bosch.[2]

c. Another group of designer drugs have a purely stimulating effect, like the amphetamine group. They include "Ice", which is smoked in the form of amphetamine crystals and produces an intense euphoria lasting at least twenty-four hours. This is of course followed by an enormous hangover, deep depression, a large chance of repeated use and so on. In other words, it is followed by addiction.

Many people also count crack in this group of designer drugs,[3] while for others crack was a drug discovered more or less by accident,[4] and consequently cannot be included amongst the designer drugs in the true sense of the word.

11

Drug use and drug addiction

As we saw in previous chapters, the use of drugs changes the interrelationship of the essential aspects of human beings. Although the effects of the different drugs are complicated, each individual drug has a particular characteristic effect. These can be described as follows.

- LSD mainly has the effect of causing the ethereal body to separate from the physical body.
- Marijuana/hashish mainly separates the astral body from the ethereal and physical body.
- The opiates, opium and morphine, separate the astral body from the ethereal and physical body to an even greater extent, while heroin and methadone also remove the Self from the other essential aspects to a large extent.
- Alcohol breaks down the organisation of the Self, so that the astral and ethereal forces are given free rein and the Self is cancelled out to a greater or lesser extent.
- Cocaine and amphetamines cause the astral body to descend powerfully into the ethereal and physical body.
- Ecstasy can cause the astral body to either "breathe out" powerfully (like marijuana/hashish) or "breathe in" (like cocaine and amphetamines).

The activity of the Self is cancelled out to a greater or lesser extent. In addition, the Self is forced to passively experience the effects created by the drugs and to look on helplessly while its foundations and instrument (the physical body, the ethereal body and astral body) become increasingly disabled after repeated use. These essential aspects increasingly exist in an uncontrolled situation, abandoned by the Self, as it were; the power of the drugs to a large extent determines the structure, movements and interrelationship of the essential aspects, and therefore takes the place of the Self. This

254 In place of the self

means that the development of the Self stagnates, and the other essential aspects become alienated and break down.

In this sense the use of drugs today is a step backwards in human development. This is very different from earlier times when man used certain drugs, after a long period of preparation, to temporarily restore the lost link with the spiritual world, or to create a stronger link with the earth by means of the drug, alcohol, in order to achieve greater independence and a new consciousness of the Self.

However, this era is past and the human constitution has changed. Rudolf Steiner discussed this after emphasizing how, in the Ancient Mysteries, man had to practise for years under the strict guidance of initiates before he could be given a particular consciousness-changing substance:[1] "The bodies of people were completely different in ancient times[2] ... (Why?) because our present intellect did not exist. People did not yet think for themselves as we do nowadays, but received their thoughts as inspirations. Just as we are conscious nowadays that we do not create the redness of the rose, but that the rose makes an impression on us, it was quite self-evident for people in those days to believe that their thoughts were inspired by the things around them. The cause of this was that bodies in those days were completely different. Even the composition of the blood was different.

... You have to understand this difference between the organism of man then and now. In that case, there will no longer be a desire to take substances in order to achieve different states of consciousness as was customary in ancient times and even in the Middle Ages." Elsewhere he wrote: "If man tries to do this again nowadays, or does this in the same way as in the past, this will result in illness."[3]

In the case of drug addiction this has a number of consequences for the user related to the general character of the addiction, in addition to the specific effects of the different drugs which have been discussed in this book.

The human soul loses the quality of patience. When a drug addict feels an irresistible desire for the drug he cannot wait, but must take the substance immediately. He cannot say to himself: O.K., I'll wait another day or a few days. He has to have it immediately. With the disappearance of patience, the sense of development also disappears after a while, in other words, the awareness that processes of change (including those in yourself) take time. The addict wants results straightaway and to be satisfied immediately. Thus in general it is very difficult for an addict to deal with feelings of displeasure, aggression, sorrow, disappointment or with tension and conflict, if they are not immediately resolved. This is a considerable obstacle in the inner process of change necessary to end the addiction.

In addition, drug addiction is an extremely egocentric activity. The addict always wants to draw substances towards him. He is always wanting, wanting, wanting. He no longer takes an interest in other people for their sake; other people are interesting in so far as they can be used to satisfy the addict's own needs. Thus drug addiction makes people increasingly selfish.

When he loses an interest in the outside world and in other people, the addict's world becomes smaller and smaller. He is imprisoned in his own world, which is totally dependent on his addiction. This is strikingly described by the criminologist, Ed Leuw: "Addiction is a psychological imprisonment used by the addict. He drastically reduces the world in which he operates. He creates and limits the territory with a strict regime of predictable events and ritual repetitions, a world in which confrontations with the uncertainties and demands of the hard outside world are restricted to a minimum."[4] As a result, he becomes increasingly isolated from his environment (friends, acquaintances, parents, members of the family, etc.), grows increasingly lonely and is ultimately left alone with his beloved (and hated) drug(s). Everything which happens in this context is actually a stagnation of his development.

In his novel, *Op de rug van vuile zwanen* (On the Back of Dirty Swans), René Stoute wrote: "The junkie is always travelling, but not really going anywhere. In his movement he stands still."[5] His development stops. In the end the only thing which is still interesting to him is the experience produced by the drugs. Apart from this, the world becomes less and less worthwhile.

Thus, for the addict, reality becomes smaller and smaller, and finally the outside world no longer reaches him. Just as a plant wilts and finally dies in the cold and dark when the light and the warmth of the sun no longer shine on it, the addict increasingly curls up in the web of addiction which he has spun himself and gets closer and closer to death.

Addiction is darkness; in William Burroughs's novel, *Junkie*, his wife tells him when she sees that he is becoming an addict again: "Don't you want to do anything? You know how terrible you are when you're addicted. It's as though all the lights go out."[6]

Often there is then a moment when the addict becomes truly aware that he is completely stuck and realizes that continuing in this way will sooner or later lead to his downfall. This moment of enlightenment can give him courage to conquer his addiction.

References

1. Introduction

1. Ministry of Public Health, Welfare and Culture, Memorandum on the problem of addiction, June 1992, p.2.
2. Including methadone addicts. Hoekstra and Derks, p.61.
3. Minjon, Wolters, p.16.
4. "In 1990 about 6% of clients who came to the consultation clinics for alcohol and drugs had problems with cannabis, amongst other things (Ladis, 1990). This is 16% of the new registered drugs clients. Almost half of these 1,095 clients came for cannabis as their primary problem." Hoekstra and Derks, p.60.
5. Hoekstra and Derks, p.66.
6. Goos, p.30.
7. Goos, p.31.
8. Schmidbauer, Vom Scheidt, p.632.
9. Regular use means that Ecstasy is taken once a month or more often, Adelaars, p.65.
10. Schmidbauer, Vom Scheidt, pp.9–10.
11. Van Epen, p.15.
12. Thus addiction is essentially quite separate from any physical dependency (habituation): for example, if the body has become dehabituated after treatment at a centre, but the desire remains and the Self is still too weak to say no, the addict is still addicted.
    Conversely, if one is able to say no to the desire, although the body is still habituated and this is achieved during and after the painful withdrawal symptoms, so that saying no means a permanent "no", the person is no longer an addict.
13. Van Epen, p.16.
14. Visser, pp.97–98.
15. Sahini, pp.17–18.

2. Historical outline of drug use

1. See Rudolf Steiner's works.
2. Quoted from Van Epen, pp.111–112.
3. Spieksma, p.9.
4. Simonis, pp.112–113.

5.   See, e.g. the gin epidemic in the 18th century described in chapter 7.
6.   Widdershoven and Ter Meulen, p.106.
7.   Hoekstra, Derks, p.58.
8.   Schmidbauer, Vom Scheidt, p.189.
9.   Schmidbauer, Vom Scheidt, p.153.
10. Simonis, p.25.
11. Simonis, p.28.
12. Simonis, p.29.
13. Schrijnemakers, pp.654–655.
14. Van Epen, p.80.
15. Van Ree, Esseveld, p.90.
16. Schultes, Hofmann, p.14.
17. Schultes, Hofmann, p.96.
18. Schultes, Hofmann, p.97.

3. The use of drugs in our time

1.   Hendriks, Molleman and Schippers, p.64.
2.   De Zwart (employee of the Dutch Institute for Alcohol and Drugs = NIAD), p.13. I am grateful to the author for making the 1989–1991 figures available to me in anticipation of a new publication.
3.   De Zwart, p.22; and data provided by the author.
4.   De Zwart, p.61; and data provided by the author.

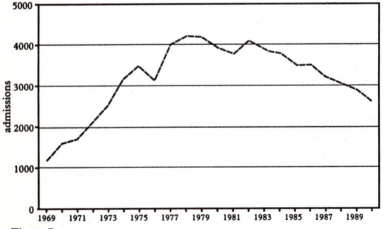

Figure 5

Hospital admissions as a result of alcohol abuse in the Netherlands 1969–1990 (De Zwart, p.36, and data made available by the author).

Table 2

Clients with alcohol and drug problems 1968–1991
(De Zwart, p.45, and data made available by the author.)

Year	Clients with alcohol problems	Clients with drug problems
1968	11,238	300
1969	11,338	635
1970	10,963	1,417
1971	9,430	2,942
1972	12,088	2,780
1973	12,456	3,330
1974	11,726	3,467
1975	12,368	4,198
1976	14,009	5,511
1977	14,064	5,983
1978	15,318	5,734
1979	16,578	5,904
1980	14,398	6,575
1981	11,826	6,786
1982	10,500	7,188
1983	13,073	8,302
1984	16,346	11,545
1985	14,476	9,492
1986	12,698	9,568
1987	13,135	9,355
1988	13,801	10,744
1989	14,649	11,949
1990	15,155	12,650
1991	14,596	13,463

5. Table 1 does not give an exact impression, but serves as an indication, as methods of collecting data have improved over the years.

6. De Zwart, p.58. See explanation with footnote 2.

7. De Zwart, p.21.

8. De Zwart, p.52; supplemented and partly amended with recent data made available to me by the author.

9. Excluding methadone addicts.

10. Many people had problems as the result of the use of drugs, as shown by:

a The great increase in the number of hospital admissions for alcohol abuse in the Netherlands between 1969 and 1990 (see fig. 5 on previous page).

b The increase in the number of clients with alcohol problems and the enormous growth in the number of clients with drug problems registered at

the Dutch consultation centres for alcohol and drugs. (See table 2 above.)
11. Van Ree, Esseveld, p.166.
12. Van Epen, pp.86–87.
13. Burroughs, pp.142–143.
14. De Loor, pp.13–14.
15. De Loor, p.15.
16. Sahini, p.7.

4. LSD

1. However, nowadays lysergic acid can also be composed entirely synthetically, although this does not detract from the following statement, as the structure of the substance found in the natural state is reproduced in the synthetic composition.
2. Schultes, Hofmann, p.102.
3. Schultes, Hofmann, pp.102–103.
4. Schultes, Hofmann, p.103.
5. Richter, pp.56–57.
6. Richter, pp.63–66.
7. Van Baaren, p.102.
8. Schmidbauer, Vom Scheidt, p.215.
9. Schmidbauer, Vom Scheidt, p.243.
10. Sarwey, p.100.
11. Quoted in Schmidbauer, Vom Scheidt, pp.214–216.
12. Cashman, p.67
13. Schmidbauer, Vom Scheidt, p.64.
14. Hiebel, p.3.
15. Quotation from a lecture by Albert Hofmann, 27 February 1970, p.61.
16. Schmidbauer, Vom Scheidt, p.240.
17. Schmidbauer, Vom Scheidt, p.239.
18. Schmidbauer, Vom Scheidt, p.241.
19. Schmidbauer, Vom Scheidt, p.237.
20. Koob, 1989, p.103. For our view on this matter, see the remainder of this chapter and chapter 11, pp.253–254.
21. Kübler-Ross, p.43.
22. Kübler-Ross, pp.46–47.
23. Van Epen, p.106.
24. Hiebel, p.2.
25. Bühler, p.33 et seq.
26. Account of a young ex-soldier in Moody, 1980, p.60.

27. Moody, 1980, p.56.

28. Kübler-Ross, pp.51–52.

29. Our ethereal body has two different components: we inherit one part from our parents, while the other part comes from the cosmic ethereal substance when we are incarnated.

30. Schmidbauer, Vom Scheidt, p.246–251.

31. Schmidbauer, Vom Scheidt, p.478–479.

32. Lievegoed 1983, p.153.

33. Schmidbauer, Vom Scheidt, p.230.

34. Schmidbauer, Vom Scheidt, p.226.

35. Lievegoed 1983, p.154.

36. Schmidbauer, Vom Scheidt, p.226.

37. Van Ree, Esseveld, p.160.

38. Schmidbauer, Vom Scheidt, p.223.

39. Van Ree, Esseveld, p.160.

40. Van Epen, pp.108–109.

41. Van Epen (pp. 105–106): "One of the peculiar properties of LSD is that it has an effect when minute quantities are taken. These quantities are calculated in micrograms; one microgram is 1/1,000 mg and 20–30 micrograms (i.e. 0.0000 to 0.00003 grammes) is sufficient to produce a clear reaction. The usual dose of a black market trip is 50–100 micrograms, but it should be remembered that only a small part of the LSD taken reaches the brain. It has been calculated that for every 3,000 brain cells there is one molecule of LSD. About 20 minutes after it is taken there is no LSD left in the brain at all; curiously the effects of the trip start after only 30 to 60 minutes."

42. Schmidbauer, Vom Scheidt p.220: "Of the LSD taken orally, very little goes into the human brain, which can be proved with radioactive marked LSD; the rest is transported primarily to the liver and kidneys and is excreted within eight to twelve hours."

43. Fromberg 1991, p.23.

44. Steiner, *Dreams, Hallucinations, Visions*, pp.31–32.

45. Koob 1990, p.184.

46. Lievegoed 1983, p.144.

47. Schmidbauer, Vom Scheidt, p.216.

48. Treichler 1981, p.214.

49. Van Epen, p.113.

50. *The Weed and the Flower*, p.35.

51. Schmidbauer, Vom Scheidt, p.432.

52. Schmidbauer, Vom Scheidt, p.216.

53. Van Epen, p.109.
54. Van Ree, Esseveld, pp.162–163.
55. Steiner, *The Science of the Secrets of the Soul*, pp.51–52.
56. *The Weed and the Flower*, p.34.
57. Steiner, *A Road to the Self-Knowledge of Man/the Threshold of the Spiritual World*, p.21.
58. Cashman, pp 96–98.
59. Cashman, pp 83–84.
60. Niederhäuser, 'LSD', p.26.
61. Cashman, p.57.
62. Van Ree, Esseveld, p.163.
63. Steiner, *A Road to the Self-Knowledge of Man/the Threshold of the Spiritual World*, p.24.
64. Bühler, pp.40–42.
65. Cashman, p.78.
66. Niederhäuser, p.28.
67. Moody 1988, p.27.
68. Moody 1988, p.25.
69. Van Epen, p.197.
70. *The Weed and the Flower*, pp.34–35.
71. Steiner, *The Science of the Secrets of the Soul*, p.72.
72. Steiner, *A Road to the Self-Knowledge of Man/the Threshold of the Spiritual World*, pp.115–116.
73. Schmidbauer, Vom Scheidt, p.278.
74. Van Baaren, p.96.
75. Schmidbauer, Vom Scheidt, p.223.
76. *The Weed and the Flower*, pp.113–115.
77. Bühler, p.32
78. Cashman, p.78.

5. Marijuana/Hashish

1. Nowadays, THC can also be produced synthetically; when it is taken the effects are virtually identical to those with the use of marijuana and hashish.
2. Schouten, p.36.
3. However, recent research has shown that male specimens also contain consciousness expanding substances, though in much smaller amounts (Segal, p.113).
4. Schouten, p.32.

5. Schouten, p.34.
6. Van Ree, Esseveld, pp.57–58.
7. Coen van Zwol in *NRC Handelsblad,* 17 February 1993.
8. Schultes, Hofmann, p.95.
9. Schultes, Hofmann, p.92.
10. Schmidbauer, Vom Scheidt, p.87.
11. Schouten, p.49.
12. M. Kooyman, p.43.
13. Schouten, p.51.
14. Schouten, p.52.
15. Schouten, p.53.
16. Schultes, Hofmann, p.101.
17. Schouten, p.58.
18. Schouten, p.61.
19. Van Epen, p.101.
20. Schultes, Hofmann, p.98.
21. Schouten, p.54.
22. Driessen, Van Dam and Olsson, pp.2–14.
23. Gunning, p.5.
24. "In addition, tar is breathed in which contains carcinogenic substances such as benzopyrees. The smoke of marijuana cigarettes contains 70% more carcinogenic substances than the smoke of tobacco … Smoking marijuana for one month is as damaging to the lungs as smoking cigarettes for a year." (Van Epen, p.100).
In addition, the immune systems which combat bacteria in the lungs are adversely affected.
25. Gunning, p.4.
26. Schmidbauer, Vom Scheidt, p.96.
27. Gunning, pp.8–9.
28. Schmidbauer, Vom Scheidt, p.97.
29. Schouten, p.122.
30. Van Epen, p.96.
31. Steiner, *Laughing and Crying.*
32. See "The effects of LSD." p.52 et seq.
33. *The Weed and the Flower,* p.55.
34. *The Weed and the Flower,* p.56.
35. Mees, 1988, p.41.
36. This seems to contradict the fact that for a number of users the effect of cannabis actually momentarily strengthens the memory. However, in our view this is caused by the fact that a certain part of the ethereal body on

which the user has focused his attention, partly separates away from the physical body, with the result that the memory content in this part of the ethereal body can correctly enter consciousness by means of a reflection which is not yet distorted, where the connection between the ethereal body and the physical body is still intact. However, there is still the danger of inner wandering, floating and confusion during the high. If it is necessary to think logically, users under the influence are unable to do so; in psychological achievement tests they perform less well than subjects who have not taken the drug. In learning activities their results are also poorer. Van Ree and Esseveld (p. 140) wrote: "Laboratory studies have shown that under the influence of cannabis the ability to learn – and in particular the ability to remember new and complicated material – deteriorates."

37.   Steiner, *Profession and Karma*, lecture, 6 Nov 1916. (Rudolf Steiner used the term "ganglion system", which was common at the beginning of this century, to indicate the autonomous/vegetative nervous system.)

38.   Schouten, p.128.

39.   Kooyman, p.59.

40.   Steiner, *The Education of the Child in the Light of Anthroposophy*.

41.   Kooyman, p.52.

42.   Van Epen, p.95.

43.   Schmidbauer, Vom Scheidt, pp.472–473.

44.   Van Epen, p.97.

45.   Burroughs, pp.31–32.

46.   Steiner, *Nature and Man seen from the Point of View of Spiritual Science*, lecture, 20 February 1924.

47.   Schmidbauer, Vom Scheidt, pp.103–104.

48.   Schmidbauer, Vom Scheidt, p.120.

49.   Bott, p.121.

50.   Van Epen, p.100.

51.   Schmidbauer, Vom Scheidt, p.119.

52.   Discussion of research by Zuckerman, Frank, Hingson et al. by Van Ingen, pp.231–232.

53.   Schmidbauer, Vom Scheidt, p.117.

54.   Van Epen, pp.100–101.

55.   Gunning, p.4. also Cohen, 1981, quoted in Segal: "THC is retained in the brain ... for a long time because of its insolubility in water."

6. Opiates

1.   Behr, p.15 et seq.

2.   Koob 1989, pp.99–100.

3.   Van Epen, pp.40–41.

4.   Behr, p.43.

5.   Behr, p.42.

6.   Behr, p.50.

7.   Behr, p.53.

8.   Schmidbauer, Vom Scheidt, p.302.

9.   Steiner, *Reflections on Spiritual Science*, lecture, 30 December 1916.

10. Johnson, p.656.

11. Johnson, p.657.

12. Behr, p.158.

13. Behr, p.121.

14. Behr, p.119.

15. Johnson, p.659.

16. Van der Meulen, p.13.

17. *Frankfurter Allgemeine Zeitung*, 19 May 1992, pp.11–12.

18. Van Epen, p.34.

19. Behr, p.100.

20. Behr, p.111.

21. Behr, p.114.

22. During the 1960s, street heroin in the United States rarely contained more than 5% diacetylmorphine. Samples sold in the streets in the Netherlands in the 1970s usually contain 20–30% pure heroin (Van Epen, p.35). Turkish heroin no. 4 ("Turkish honey") can contain up to 90% diacetylmorphine (Schmidbauer, Vom Scheidt, p.307).

23. Schmidbauer, Vom Scheidt, pp.302–303, Koob 1990, pp.219–221.

24. Treichler, p.23.

25. Steiner, Wegman, chapter 1.

26. Steiner, *Spiritual Science and Medicine*, p.331.

27. Schmidbauer, Vom Scheidt, p.315.

28. Schmidbauer, Vom Scheidt, pp.314–315.

29. Bott, p.92.

30. Schmidbauer, Vom Scheidt, p.310.

31. Normally these (opiate) receptors are taken over by so-called enkephalins under certain circumstances such as pain, fear, shock, etc. i.e. by substances in the body with a chemical structure which is very similar to the structure of opiates (S. Snyder. p.146 and 154). These enkephalins take over the enkephalin or opiate receptors, when the astral body withdraws from the nervous system under the above-mentioned circumstances so that man enters a state of anaesthesis or slight (astral) separation.

32. According to S. Snyder, the so-called peri-aquaductal grey area in the

central brain and certain parts (particularly the central part) of the thalamus are of essential importance for the perception of pain in this context (pp. 100–101).

33. Schmidbauer, Vom Scheidt, pp.310–311.

34. Obviously not with the opiate receptors which are also there.

35. Steiner, *Nature and Man from the Point of View of Spiritual Science,* lecture, 20 February 1924.
This is wrong – as we already saw with the effect of marijuana/hashish – partly because of the partial separation of the ethereal body from the physical body so that experiences in the astral world are distorted in the "distorting mirror of consciousness." Also see "The effects of LSD", p.52 et seq.

36. Schmidbauer, Vom Scheidt, p.314.

37. Steiner, *The Science of the Secrets of the Soul,* chapter 2, p.55.

38. For the relationship between the ethereal body and the memory see page. 55 et seq.

39. Steiner, *Historical Observation,* lecture, 14 January. 1917.

40. Steiner, *Life of Man and Earth,* lecture, 18 April 1923.

41. Steiner, *Spiritual Science of Man,* lecture, 2 November 1908.

42. In this sense opium is more dangerous than LSD because, in the case of addiction, opium is used virtually continuously and the memory is therefore completely overburdened. LSD provides a more waking "dream consciousness" (caused by the partial separation of the ethereal body from the physical body) and is used much less frequently partly because it does not cause physical dependency in contrast with opium.

43. These feelings follow the unpleasant experiences for the user taking opium for the first time – caused by its toxic character – such as nausea, dizziness and vomiting (see nicotine, alcohol, etc). After continued use these effects disappear.

44. Steiner, *Historical Observation,* lecture, 14 January 1917.

45. Rudolf Steiner: "At the time that his Self was torn away, his memory was intact", lecture, 14 January 1917.

46. Hessenbruch, p.15.

47. Hessenbruch, pp.8–9.

48. There is a change in the enkephalin metabolism in the nervous system caused by opium which causes the production of enkephalin to stagnate as the enkephalin receptors are taken up by opiates during the state of intoxication.

49. Koob, 1990, p.221.

50. Thus there is the stagnating enkephalin metabolism in parts of the nervous system. During the state of intoxication the enkephalin receptors are taken up by opiates so that when this state comes to an end and the opiates have abandoned these receptors, the enkephalin receptors can no

longer be taken up by encephalins as they are no longer being produced. Thus, instead of enkephalin metabolism there is an artificial opiate metabolism, and if no opiates are administered, the body can no longer function "normally."

51. Hessenbruch, pp.15–16.

52. For detailed description of the effects of heroin, see p.148 et seq.

53. The text reads literally: "some examples" rather than "one example." However, we quote only one example.

54. Van Epen, pp.15–16.

55. Below there is a characterization of the literature. The authors mentioned build on a basic knowledge of Spiritual Science (Anthroposophy) which is presumed to be familiar to the readers, as indicated in the main works by Rudolf Steiner.

The unearthly paradisiacal atmosphere which the opium user enters
H. Pelikan, *Knowledge of Healing Plants*, Part II:
After describing the characteristic growth, flowering and propagation of *Papaver somniferum*, Pelikan describes that the toxic milky sap from which opium is prepared is a "remnant" of the old so-called Lemurian evolutionary period of the earth, i.e. the time before the Fall when man still lived in the state of consciousness which existed in paradise. The use of opium evokes this ancient state of consciousness.

In his book, *Plants: A Road to Understanding Your Essence*, Parts I and II, Gerbert Grohmann also explores this theme, and in particular describes the link between this milky sap and his so-called Old Moon phase of the earth (the former planetary embodiment of our planet prior to the earth), in which the Lemurian stage of the earth can be seen as a metamorphosed repetition of this Old Moon phase. The use of opium takes man back to this distant, ancient, dreamlike state of consciousness of the Old Moon time in a way that is very destructive for him.

In *Life Processes in Nature*, Jochem Bockemühl not only describes the way in which *Papaver somniferum* grows and flowers above the earth, but also describes the underground growth of the roots which can be observed in a particular way.

In this respect it is striking that the formation of the roots, which is very minimal anyway, quickly stops at the moment that the plant uses its forces in the sap, in particular for the development of the milky sap of the ovary. At that moment it is as though the plant draws back into the earth.

Forgetting and Remembering
I will describe this in more detail, because the effect that opium both produces oblivion and stimulates the memory, is reminiscent of ancient times when man underwent processes in the Mysteries as an initiate which achieved the same result. This is why opium possibly played a role in these Mysteries as one of the ingredients of the so-called drink of oblivion, as described in the section on the history of opium. Because I consider that

this is one of the root causes of the use of drugs, i.e. to change consciousness by means of a physical substance, I will quote in detail some of the passages from two lectures by Rudolf Steiner in which he wrote in very concrete terms about the knowledge of the Ancient Mysteries and about ancient and new initiation methods (published under the title: *Ancient and New Initiation Methods*, lectures, 1 February 1922 and 12 February 1922). Again we should remember that Rudolf Steiner is developing a basic anthroposophical knowledge which is presumed to be familiar to the reader.

I quote (11 February 1922): "It can be ... extremely elucidating to observe something which was considered a matter of great importance in the various Mystery sites. Certainly, the preparations and subsequent tests etc. which the pupils of the Mysteries, the initiates, had to undergo, differed from one site to another. However, the differences are only like those which apply when a mountain is climbed from different sides to reach the same summit by different means. Ultimately everything led to a single goal in the Mysteries.

"No matter how different things were then, it is possible to indicate two aspects of these Mysteries to which everyone had to subject themselves, as the main thing. There was the so-called intoxication of oblivion, and secondly, something within the Mysteries which had the effect of a huge shock or the experience of great fear. These two things can no longer be experienced in the same ways nowadays to obtain higher extrasensory insights. Nowadays, everything has to be experienced in a spiritual way, while the pupils of the Ancient Mysteries experienced things in such a way that they always needed physical help. Something similar happens, though the difference is that in this present spiritual quest for higher knowledge everything is in the sphere of consciousness, while in the past it fell under the sphere of instinctive, dreamlike states. Because something like the intoxication of oblivion was presented in all the Mysteries, bringing about something like a physical shock, man was actually overcome with regard to his external intellectualism, even if this was duller than it is now, but it still controlled him with regard to his relationship with the external world.

"Thus man was brought into a dull life both by means of the intoxication of oblivion and by the other means, which can be compared with shock and the arousal of fear.

"What was the meaning of the intoxication of oblivion? The important thing was not that things were forgotten. Certainly things were forgotten as a result of this intoxication, but the effect which it had was produced because the initiate was baptised in a certain ceremony, prepared in a particular way and certain measures were taken before he was given the drink. It was a purely physical drink, which meant that because of the way in which it was given, man forgot his life from birth. This is something that can once again be achieved by means of the development of the soul and the spirit, although it is achieved nowadays by first evoking a clear consciousness of the tableaux of life, comprising everything from birth. This is then suppressed, and in this way man enters the spiritual path of his life before birth or before conception. The same thing was achieved in a more physical way by means of the ancient intoxication of oblivion.

"However, the essential point is not that man forgets, for a negative condition is never the essential point. The positive thing that was achieved by this is that thoughts became more mobile and intense, though they also became duller. They became dreamy precisely because the physical organism was touched. The effect of this intoxication of oblivion on the physical organism can be described very precisely – the brain becomes more liquid, as it were, than it is in ordinary life. Because the brain becomes more liquid, and man therefore thought more with brain water than with the solid matter of the brain, his thoughts became more mobile and intense.

Nowadays, this must be achieved by a direct method, viz. by the development of the soul and the spirit as described in *The Path to an Insight to a Higher Region* and in *The Science of the Secrets of the Soul*. However, in those times the brain was made more liquid by outside influences. This means that man's spiritual essence, as it was before man was connected to a physical body in conception, can once again penetrate the brain as it did in the spiritual world. This is the essence... I would say that the constitution of the brain now is such that the eternal aspect of man cannot become conscious in the brain. Because of this, external impressions are able to enter. When man received the intoxication of oblivion, he was able to take into the brain that which was present as a spiritual quality before conception or before birth. This is one aspect.

"The other aspect was mentioned above: man experienced a sort of shock. What happens when a person has a shock? He goes stiff, and the shock can be so great that this stiffness affects the whole person. A normal person can walk round in ordinary life, while the rigid cataleptic person cannot walk because his muscles are too stiff. In a person who is not rigid the body takes in this eternal aspect. The spiritual, eternal aspect is taken into the blood and muscles. Therefore it cannot be perceived; it cannot enter the brain because it is taken in below, and so it cannot be perceived, but is released freely and independently when the muscles become rigid.

This rigidity of the muscles was caused by the effect of the shock. Therefore the spiritual quality was not taken into the rest of the organism, except the brain, but was released. As a result man had a spiritual quality in the brain because his brain had become weak and soft with the intoxication of oblivion and because the rest of the organism was prevented from taking in the spiritual quality. This means that the spiritual quality was perceived.

"... I would expressly point out that these things cannot be imitated nowadays. People would not know how to do this now and it would not suit them. Nowadays, everything should be achieved through spiritual means."

In the lecture he gave a day later (12 February 1922) Rudolf Steiner summarized the above again, adding another aspect: "I said that the two essential things which were important in the Ancient Mysteries were the intoxication of oblivion, on the one hand, and producing states of fearful, frightening shock, on the other. The intoxication of oblivion certainly made man erase the memory of everything which had taken place in his life on earth. However, I said that this negative aspect was not the main point; the main point was that during the process of knowledge of the Mysteries the brain was in a sense actually made weak and soft, and therefore the spiritual matter which would otherwise have been repelled, was not repelled by the brain, but entered it, so that man became aware of it as a result: yes, I have an eternal spiritual soul which was there before my birth and before my conception.

"The other point is that the rest of the organism became rigid as a result of a shock. However, when an organism is rigid it does not draw up spiritual matter as it does normally, insofar as this is expressed by the will. It is as though the rigidified body withdraws from the spiritual matter, on the one hand, while, on the other hand, this spiritual matter becomes perceptible. The conceptual side of the spiritual matter became visible to the pupils of the Ancient Mysteries because the brain was softer. The will became perceptible because the rest of the organ rigidified. In this way the initiation gave man an idea of his spiritual essence. However, this idea had a completely dreamlike character. What was it really which was released, on the one hand, in ideas, and on the other hand, in the will? It was that which descends from the spiritual world and connects with man's physical body ... Yesterday I said that if man wished to do this again nowadays or wants to do this in the same way as in the past, this would produce a spiritual condition."

56.   Burroughs, p.20.

57.   Behr, p.139.

58.   Behr, p.144.

59.   Stoute, pp.22–23.

60.   Zeylmans van Emmichoven, p.128.

61.   Van Epen, p.37.

62.   Van Epen, pp.36–37.

63.   "As a result of cramps at the stomach exit, the passage from the stomach to the intestine can be obstructed for a long time. In suicide attempts with opiates taken orally this is often of life-saving importance; the poison can be pumped out of the stomach many hours after it has been taken ...

"Cramps of the musculature of the gall bladder and gall passages may be similar to a 'gall stone attack' in heroin addicts; many have been unnecessarily operated on. Cramp in the involuntary muscle of the bladder often makes it difficult for heroin or methadone addicts to urinate; nurses on methadone programmes know about this. They often find it difficult to make patients pass water in time." (Van Epen, pp.36–37).

64.   Behr, p.143.

Obviously neurological processes also take place in the system governing the metabolism and the limbs. Zeylmans van Emmichoven (p. 127): "It is clear that the three systems of organs interpenetrate. In the nervous-sensory system, metabolism is as necessary as the relationship with rhythmic processes ... On the other hand, in the organs belonging to the metabolic system, the rhythmic and neurological processes interact only mildly."

65. In addition, the respiratory centre is inhibited. This respiratory centre can be seen as a physical reflection of the respiratory process in the lungs and the stimulation or inhibition of this respiratory centre affects the respiration of the lungs. Cf. Walter Holtzapfel in *Im Kraftfeld der Organe* (In the Force Field of the Organs) (p. 25): "Thirst comes from the liver. The so-called thirst centre in the mid-brain is a reflection of this liver function."

66. Van Epen, p.36.

67. Behr, p.146.

68. Stoute, pp.22–23.

69. The blood has a curious place in relation to these three systems. It constantly flows through the whole organism, thus connecting different organ systems. The blood could be described as a fourth organ system which makes the previous three into a unity. This immediately suggests a comparison with the place of the "Self" amongst the three groups of spiritual functions in which thought, feelings and the will manifest themselves. Just as the manifestation of the Self accompanies all other manifestations, including those of the feelings and the will, it could be said that each organ function is ultimately connected to the blood processes which flow through the entire organ, linking everything. (Zeylmans van Emmichoven in *The Human Soul* [pp. 129–130].)

70. Behr, p.146.

71. Stoute, pp.55–56.

72. Behr, pp.143, 146, 147 and 145.

73. Schmidbauer, Vom Scheidt, p.314.

74. Koob 1990, p.227.

75. Van Ree, Esseveld, p.84.

76. Behr, p.9 et seq.

77. Koob, 1989, pp.99–100.

78. Visser, p.114.

79. Schmidbauer, Vom Scheidt, p.317.

80. Van Ree, Esseveld, p.74.

81. Visser, p.94.

82. Van Ree, Esseveld, p.76.

83. Schmidbauer, Vom Scheidt, p.318.

84. Burroughs, pp.104–108.

85. Van Epen, p.47.

86. Van Epen, p.48.

87. Van Ree, Esseveld, p.226.

88. Research by F. Bschor, H.G. Schommer and J. Wessel discussed by Swierstra, p.88.

89. Swierstra, pp.78–92.

90. Schmidbauer, Vom Scheidt, p.345.

7. Alcohol

1. Schmidbauer, Vom Scheidt, p.84.

2. Data made available by W.M. de Zwart (NIAD).

3. Hendriks, Molleman and Schippers, p.64.

4. Data made available by W.M. de Zwart (NIAD).

5. Spieksma, p.10.

6. De Zwart, pp.34–35; plus data made available by the author.

7. De Zwart, p.30.

8. De Zwart, p.33.

9. De Zwart, p.25.

10. Minjon, Wolters, p.14.

11. De Zwart, p.48.

12. Schmidbauer, Vom Scheidt, p.23.

13. Schmidbauer, Vom Scheidt, p.59.

14. Steiner, *Lectures on the Gospel According to St. John*, lecture, 23 May 1908.

15. Simonis, pp.99–100.

16. Simonis, p.105.

17. "For example, in his *Laws*, Plato's contributors to the dialogue explain the educational aspects of drinking wine, even with the aim of introducing the drinking of wine by the State as a means of assessing and practising the control of the desires and self-discipline. In the discussions he also draws up laws for the drinkers 'to ensure that the optimistic and foolhardy drinker who becomes more exuberant than he should, and is not prepared to be moderate or to be silent, talk, drink or sing when it is his turn, is now forced to do exactly the opposite'." (Preiser, p.302).

18. Legnaro, p.88 (Rolleston 1933, "Alcoholism in Medieval England". In: *The British Journal of Inebriety* 31 (2): 33–49).

19. Legnaro, pp.87–88.

20. Legnaro, p.89.

21. Legnaro, p.86.

22. Legnaro, p.90.

23. Stolleis, p.101.

24. Aldo Legnaro, p.91.

25. Stolleis, pp.102–103.

26. Legnaro, p.92.

27. Coffey, pp.106–107.

28. Legnaro, pp.92–93.

29. Van Amerongen, p.31.

30. Legnaro, p.93, on birthdays, at weddings, christenings, communions, etc.

31. Vogt, p.115.

32. This had catastrophic consequences for the social structures of many African tribes and nations who had little or no contact with alcohol (some nations did use a weak alcoholic drink in their religious rituals, though this had a much lower alcohol percentage than the imported distilled alcohol from Europe). Albert Schweitzer described how countless settlements and villages simply disappeared as a result of alcohol. Van Epen wrote: "The colonists 'bought' raw materials, goods, artefacts and manpower and 'paid' with alcohol, particularly with very strong distilled drinks of inferior quality. This resulted in an extremely high percentage of alcoholics among the negro population and the side-effects of high levels of aggression, suicide, physical illness, psychosis, etc. ... Curiously the negroes had had an alcohol culture for many centuries; several sorts of palm wine had been around since time immemorial. However, there was a lengthy ritual related to this weak alcoholic drink which imposed all sorts of restrictions on the user and actually allowed him to drink the wine only on certain festive occasions and in a particular social context. However, the spirits imported by the white man fell completely outside this ritual and had a totally different function for the population, viz. that of a narcotic and stimulant. It was many generations before the negro population learnt to live with the new drug and meanwhile a great deal of damage had been done." (J.H. Van Epen, p.169).

33. Van Amerongen, p.36.

34. Exceptions to this were France and Italy where the consumption of alcohol fell in the 1970s, a decline which continued in the 1980s.

35. Hansen, p.71.

36. Feest, pp.164, 166.

37. Feest, p.163.

38. Schmidbauer, Vom Scheidt, p.51.

39. Levine, p.119; Widdershoven and Ter Meulen, p.106.

40. Levine, p.119.

41. Levine, p.121.

42. Levine, p.120.

43. There was also a much smaller and more moderate temperance

movement which was primarily aimed at reducing the consumption of spirits. Beer and wine were considered less dangerous. The main aim was not total abstinence but the reduction of excessive alcohol consumption. It was an appeal to common sense.

44.   Levine, pp.126–127.

45.   Levine, p.127.

46.   Levine, p.130.

47.   While the grapes ripen, the spores of the yeast in the flesh of the grapes also form a little bit of alcohol. Kaspar Hauser who had been locked up on his own in a virtually dark room for ten years from his earliest youth was extremely sensitive to this shortly after his release (as he was to all other sensory impressions): "It was not only the smell of alcohol which evoked symptoms of inebriation in him – swaying and slurring – but also eating grapes or drinking a few drops of grape juice." (Van Manen, p.47).

48.   Yeast spores are extremely primitive, pointed fungi, which, like all fungi, break down organic substances so that they eventually become minerals.

49.   I have not discussed the other details and technical aspects of wine making as I am solely concerned here with the principle of the formation of alcohol.

50.   The term "malt" describes the grain which has been artificially germinated. Then the process is suddenly terminated (growth forces are released so that the fermentation is optimal) and the germinated grains are removed.

51.   Schmidbauer, Vom Scheidt, p.97.

52.   Buddecke, pp.472–473; interview with H.H. Vogel and Weirauch, p.68.

53.   Segal, pp.258, 259. These data are based on a body weight of 75 kg in a person who is not addicted to alcohol. In general, excessive drinkers and alcoholics can tolerate higher percentages: "The highest part per thousand ever measured was 15 parts per thousand. This was in a 24-year-old American alcoholic who did not die as a result." (Spieksma p.15).

54.   Bott, p.15.

55.   Lievegoed, p.154.

56.   Steiner, *Nature and Man from the Point of View of Spiritual Science*, lecture, 20 February 1924.

57.   Renzenbrink, p.57.

58.   Pelikan, p.116.

59.   Steiner, Wegman, chapter 8.

60.   Spieksma, pp.30–31; Geerlings and Wolters, pp.79–80.

61.   Spieksma, p.31.

62.   Spieksma, p.30. In general, alcoholics do not eat much, so that the conversion of carbohydrates into blood sugar from food hardly takes place.

In addition, the breakdown of glycogen in the liver to blood sugar is often impossible because the supplies of glycogen are (virtually) exhausted.

63. Spieksma, p.31. This is sometimes explained by the fact that in alcoholics there are higher levels of blood plasma, cortisol and adrenaline. (Cortisol and adrenaline mobilize glucose from its storage place if there is any glycogen available in the tissue).

64. As, for example, in the case of reduced secretion of insulin and insulin resistance. (Insulin converts blood sugar to glycogen; this then takes place to a lesser extent so that more blood sugar circulates.) Research by Singh, Kumar, Snyder, Ellyin and Gilders, discussed by Smal, p.123.

65. Van Epen, pp.170–171.

66. Steiner, *Nature and Man from the Point of View of Spiritual Science*, lecture, 19 January 1924.

67. Van Epen, p.171.

68. "It can also be said that *life* is the characteristic of the ethereal body, *consciousness* of the astral body and *the memory* of the Self." (Rudolf Steiner, *The Science of the Secrets of the Soul*), chapter 2, p.55).

69. Steiner, *The Education of the Child in the light of Anthroposophy.*

70. Steiner, *Nature and Man from the Point of View of Spiritual Science*, lecture, 16 February 1924.

71. Weirauch, pp.18–19.

72. There may be visual hallucinations, such as small scurrying creatures in large numbers, e.g. mice, fish, cats, dogs, insects, or imaginary animals, which rise up as a result of the ethereal forces released in the organs (see LSD).

73. Spieksma, p.65.

74. Treichler, p.243.

75. Treichler, pp.244–245.

76. Research by Eagon, Porter, Van Thiel discussed by Smals, p.122.

77. Van Epen, p.181.

78. Smals, p.122.

79. Spieksma, pp.59–60.

80. Research by Mendelson and Mello, and research by Hugues, Coste, Perret, Jayle, Sebaoun, Modigliani discussed by Smals, p.122.

81. Minjon, Wolters, p.35.

82. Geerlings, p.63; Tholen, Siero and Kok, p.46.

83. Spieksma, p.59.

84. Spieksma, p.58.

85. Spieksma, p.59. As long as people drink alcohol, the FAS symptoms will appear. Even in ancient Carthage there was a law which prohibited women from drinking alcohol on their honeymoon (Spieksma, p.10).

86.   Spieksma, p.47.

87.   Van Epen, p.181.

88.   Research by Rimm, Giovannucci, Willett et al. discussed by Van Ingen, 1992, pp.34–35.

89.   Van Epen, p.182.

90.   Minjon, Wolters, p.35.

91.   Van Epen, p.183.

8. Cocaine and Amphetamines

1.   Springer, p.15 (Garcilasso de la Vega, quoted in S. Freud, *Uber Coca*).

2.   Springer, pp.15–16.

3.   Springer, pp.16–17.

4.   Schmidbauer, Vom Scheidt, p.189.

5.   Springer, p.17.

6.   Springer, p.17 – slightly abbreviated quotation.

7.   Ashley, pp.5–6.

8.   Ashley, p.9.

9.   Schmidbauer, Vom Scheidt, p.190.

10.   Van Epen, p.84.

11.   Ashley, p.11, on the basis of the literature reviewed by him, and Schmidbauer, Vom Scheidt, p.196.

12.   E. Brecher quoted by Van Epen, p.85.

13.   Schmidbauer, Vom Scheidt, pp.195–196.

14.   Schmidbauer, Vom Scheidt, p.196.

15.   Springer, p.28 (quotation from: *Coca, Detroit Therapeutic Gazette*, Vol. 5, 1881).

16.   Springer, p.30.

17.   Springer, p.37.

18.   Springer, p.36.

19.   Schmidbauer, Vom Scheidt, p.682.

20.   Schmidbauer, Vom Scheidt, p.684.

21.   Schmidbauer, Vom Scheidt, p.698.

22.   Schmidbauer, Vom Scheidt, p.685.

23.   Schmidbauer, Vom Scheidt, p.192.

24.   Schmidbauer, Vom Scheidt, p.685.

25.   Ashley, p.67.

26.   Springer, p.42.

27.   Springer, p.58.

28. Springer, pp.81–82.

29. For example, in 1923 it was estimated that there were 5–6,000 cocaine addicts in Berlin (Springer, p.78).

30. Van Epen, p.88.

31. Springer, p.188.

32. Schmidbauer, Vom Scheidt, p.201.

33. Schmidbauer, Vom Scheidt, p.200.

34. Cocaine brings about a change of the metabolic processes in the brain. For example, there is an increased effect of the neurotransmitters, noradrenaline (norapinafrine) and dopamine, in view of the fact that the re-uptake of these neurotransmitters is inhibited in the nerve ends by the effect of cocaine (Van Ree, p.45–46 and Segal, pp.147–148, 155).

35. Vom Scheidt, p.399.

Van Ree and Esseveld (p. 97): "When it is injected into the veins, this can result in spontaneous explosive orgasms though these are usually experienced as being very unpleasant." And Springer (p. 102): "Following an intravenous injections, 10 of the 20 men interviewed in a study said that they had an erection immediately after the injection. In two of these this led to an extremely painful prolonged erection which lasted for more than 24 hours."

The anaesthetizing effect of cocaine can also inhibit orgasm (e.g. by rubbing it on the head of the penis). Van Ree and Esseveld (p. 97). "Some users say that sex is fantastic after cocaine ... Cocaine prolongs the sexual act. The orgasm is delayed, but it has an extremely intense character."

South American Indians were aware of this property. Springer (p. 95): "The aphrodisiac use of the drug was certainly initially related to religious ceremonies: the collector of coca leaves had to sleep with a woman the night before the harvest in order to appease "Mama Coca." For this person, saliva containing cocaine or a cocaine infusion was rubbed on the head of the penis in order to prolong the sexual act, before the erotic adventures which took place for this goddess.

36. Van Epen, p.86.

37. Schmidbauer, Vom Scheidt, p.200.

38. Van Epen, p.87.

39. Jamin, p.168.

40. Minjon, Wolters, p.177.

41. Bieleman, Bosma, Swierstra, p.12.

42. Van Ree, Esseveld, p.97.

43. A. Conan Doyle, "The Sign of Four", in *The Collected Sherlock Holmes*.

44. Schmidbauer, Vom Scheidt, p.197.

45. Van Epen, p.86.

46. Van Ree, Esseveld, p.95.

47.   Schmidbauer, Vom Scheidt, p.201.

48.   Segal, p.77.

49.   "The spiritual yearning (craving) for the drug, and particularly for more of the drug, can be infinite. It is this craving which is seen as the core around which a far-reaching psychological addiction to cocaine can develop. When you ask an opiate addict the difference, he will say that he really needs heroin and/or methadone but does not really need cocaine, though despite this, he keeps getting coke once he has started. In this respect, it is an intensely psychologically addictive drug." (Bieleman, Bosma and Swierstra, pp.12–13).

50.   Van Ree and Esseveld, p.100.

51.   Van den Berg, p.55.

52.   Van den Berg, p.52.

53.   Treichler, 1981, p.75.

54.   Bott, p.116.

55.   However, the kidneys can also release ethereal forces. As revealed by the fact that a "cocaine psychosis can be very similar to an acute paranoid schizophrenic psychosis, with the difference that there is some awareness that the cocaine is the cause of the condition." (Van Epen, p.90). For the relationship between the kidneys and schizophrenic psychosis, see p.63 et seq.
The release of ethereal forces from the heart and lungs is also clear from the fact that an overdose can result in death from heart failure (as a result of the toxic effect on the cardiac muscles), or as a result of respiratory failure.

56.   Van Epen, p.90. In this depression there may also be damage to the liver (see p.193).

57.   Sahini, p.43.

58.   Segal, p.77.

59.   Geerlings, p.122.

60.   Geerlings, pp.122–123.

61.   Researched by Zuckerman, Frank, Hingson et al., discussed by Van Ingen, pp.231–232.

62.   Sahini, pp.44–45.

63.   Segal, pp.77–78.

64.   Springer, p.186 (quotation from L.S. Goodman, A. Gilman, Pharmacological Basis of Therapeutics, 1975).

65.   Van Epen, pp.78–79.

66.   Hyperactive children who are easily distracted.

67.   Schmidbauer, Vom Scheidt, p.371.

68.   Van Epen, p.79.

69.   Springer, p.197.

70. Springer, pp.195–197.

71. Steiner, *The Science of the Secrets of the Soul,* chapter 3, pp.74–77.

72. In addition, as described for the effects of marijuana/hashish, there may also be a connection between part of the astral body and the nervous system of the spinal cord upon falling asleep. Rudolf Steiner, *Profession and Karma,* lecture, 6 November 1916.

73. Van Ree, Esseveld, p.94. Van Epen also mentions loss of hair (p. 81).

74. Van Epen, p.81.

75. Van Ree, Esseveld, p.92.

76. Schmidbauer, Vom Scheidt, p.373.

77. This degeneration of the organization of the Self is also revealed in the rise of the blood sugar level caused by a moderate to high dose of speed. (cf. "Alcohol", p.183 et seq).

78. Van Epen, p.79.

9. Ecstasy (XTC)

1. Adelaars, pp.12–13.

2. Safrol oil is found in sassafras, parsley seed, dill, calamus, saffron and vanilla as well as nutmeg (Adelaars, p.117). Much of the XTC which was sold in the Netherlands in the late 1980s was produced using this method.

3. Adelaars, pp.20–21.

4. Adelaars, p.20 and Fromberg 1990, p.151.

5. Adelaars, p.21.

6. Adelaars, p.22.

7. Fromberg 1991, pp.5–6.

8. Fromberg, 1990, p.151.

9. Adelaars, pp.26–28.

10. Adelaars, p.27.

11. Adelaars, p.31.

12. Adelaars, p.33.

13. Fromberg 1991, p.81.

14. Fromberg 1991, pp.81–82 ("From an unpublished lecture by p.Meyer at the study conference on XTC", 23 January 1990, Amsterdam).

15. Adelaars, pp.35–38.

16. Adelaars, p.46.

17. Adelaars, p.66.

18. Adelaars, p.65.

19. Folder "XTC" compiled by the Drugs Advice Bureau, August De Loor, Amsterdam, commissioned by the Dutch Institute for Alcohol and Drugs (NIAD 1990).

20.   Adelaars, p.91.
21.   Adelaars, p.90.
22.   Adelaars, p.78.
23.   Adelaars, p.75.
24.   Fromberg 1991, p.9.
25.   Fromberg 1990, p.152.
26.   Adelaars, pp.79–80.
27.   Fromberg, 1991, p.10.
28.   Adelaars, p.74.
29.   Adelaars, pp.80–81.
30.   Adelaars, pp.81–82.
31.   Adelaars, p.96.
32.   Korf et al, 1991, pp.73–74.
33.   Korf et al, 1991, p.75.
34.   Adelaars, p.71.
35.   Adelaars, pp.94–95.
36.   Adelaars, pp.95–96.
37.   Adelaars, p.72.
38.   Adelaars, p.82.
39.   Adelaars, p.70.
40.   Adelaars, p.83.
41.   Adelaars, pp.127–133.
42.   Adelaars, pp.112–113, 127–133.
43.   Adelaars, p.113.
44.   Adelaars, pp.68–69.
45.   Fromberg 1991, pp.11–13.
46.   Adelaars, p.107.
47.   Korf et al 1991, chapter 9.
48.   Adelaars, p.111.

10. Designer drugs

1.   Schmidbauer, Vom Scheidt, p.636.
2.   Schmidbauer, Vom Scheidt, pp.336–337.
3.   Including Sahini, p.34.
4.   Including Schmidbauer, Vom Scheidt, p.636.

11. Drug use and drug addiction

1.   Steiner, *The Consciousness of Initiates*, lecture, 14 August 1924.

2. "Even during the Chaldean era" (Rudolf Steiner, same lecture). This means at the time of the so-called Chaldean era, which lasted approximately up to the beginning of the Greek culture.

3. See Opiates, footnote 55, p.267.

4. Leuw, p.186.

5. Stoute, p.24.

6. Burroughs, p.121; italics R.D.

Appendix

The UK and USA statistics given below offer some comparison to those given in the main text.

1. Introduction

a. In England in any one year, for the period 1991–93, at least 3m people took an illegal drug. In 1993 the number of addicts notified to the Home Office in England was over 25,000 (for opiates/opiods and cocaine). (Source: *Tackling Drugs Together*, HMSO Cm 2678, 1994)

b. England:

Cannabis is the most widely used illegal drug in England. (Source: *Tackling Drugs Together*, HMSO Cm 2678, 1994)
USA:

Marijuana use in the USA by age and sex for the total population

age *rate estimates*	ever used	used in past year	used in past month
12–17	10.6%	8.1%	4.0%
male	11.6	8.7	4.6
female	9.6	7.5	3.5
18–25	48.1	22.7	11.0
male	49.7	27.1	14.5
female	46.6	18.4	7.5
26–34	58.6	14.3	8.2
male	64.3	18.9	11.0
female	52.9	9.9	5.5
35+	24.8	3.3	1.6
male	31.2	4.5	2.3
female	19.2	2.2	1.0
total	**32.8**	**8.5**	**4.4**
male	**38.0**	**10.8**	**5.9**
female	**28.0**	**6.3**	**2.9**

age	ever used	used in past year	used in past month
population estimates in thousands			
12–17	2,199	1,676	838
male	1,229	916	487
female	970	760	351
18–25	13,456	6,342	3,066
male	6,831	3,720	1,998
female	6,625	2,622	1,068
26–34	22,376	5,481	3,140
male	12,114	3,555	2,074
female	10,262	1,926	1,066
35+	29,494	3,901	1,906
male	17,356	2,496	1,281
female	12,138	1,405	625
total	**67,525**	**17,400**	**8,950**
male	**37,531**	**10,687**	**5,839**
female	**29,994**	**6,713**	**3,111**

(Source: *National Household Survey on Drug Abuse: Population Estimates 1992*, US Dept. of Health and Human Services, Public Health Service).

c. USA:

Tranquillizer use in the USA by sex and age groups for the total population

age	ever used	used in past year	used in past month
rate estimates			
12–17	1.6%	1.0%	0.2%
male	1.5	0.9	0.1
female	1.6	1.2	0.2
18–25	6.8	3.0	0.6
male	7.8	3.5	0.4
female	5.8	2.6	0.8
26–34	9.0	2.0	0.5
male	10.6	2.0	0.4
female	7.4	1.9	0.6
35+	4.1	1.0	0.3
male	4.4	1.3	0.3
female	3.9	0.8	0.3
total	**5.1**	**1.5**	**0.4**
male	**5.8**	**1.7**	**0.3**
female	**4.6**	**1.3**	**0.4**

age	ever used	used in past year	used in past month
population estimates in thousands			
12–17	322	208	34
male	156	91	10
female	166	117	24
18–25	1,891	852	165
male	1,070	479	51
female	822	373	114
26–34	3,421	746	206
male	1,995	378	81
female	1,426	368	124
35+	4,920	1,241	364
male	2,463	723	166
female	2,457	518	198
total	**10,555**	**3,046**	**769**
male	**5,683**	**1,670**	**308**
female	**4,871**	**1,376**	**461**

(Source: *National Household Survey on Drug Abuse: Population Estimates 1992*, US Dept. of Health and Human Services, Public Health Service).

d. In 1988 in England, an estimated 90,000 deaths were attributable to smoking. (Source: Dept. of Health Statistics on Smoking, 1974 to 1993)

e. In the UK in 1993 the number of notified drug addicts taking cocaine was 2,463. (Source: *Tackling Drugs Together*, HMSO Cm 2678, 1994)

f. In England, police seizures of Ecstasy in 1992 involved 350,000 doses – a 300% increase on 1991. (Source: *Tackling Drugs Together*, HMSO Cm 2678, 1994)

3. The use of drugs in our time

a. USA:

Per capita ethanol consumption, 1935–1992

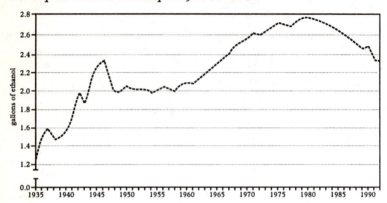

(Source: US Dept of Health and Human Services, National Institute on Alcohol Abuse and Alcoholism, Surveillance Report #31, 1994)

b. UK:

UK consumption of alcohol per head of population aged 15 and over

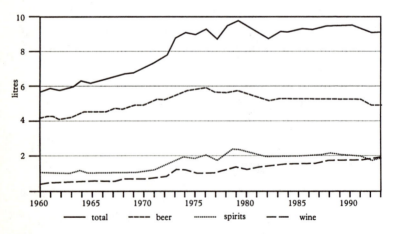

(Source: *Brewers' Society Statistical Handbook no.25,* drawing on figures from H.M. Customs and Excise and Office of Population Censuses and Surveys)

USA:
Per capita ethanol consumption by beverage type, 1977–1992

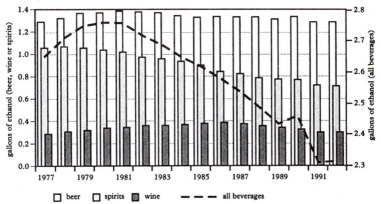

(Source: US Dept of Health and Human Services, National Institute on Alcohol Abuse and Alcoholism, Surveillance Report #31, 1994)

c. UK

Percentages exceeding sensible and safe amounts

	Men					Women				
	1984	1986	1988	1990	1992	1984	1986	1988	1990	1992
percentage who drank more than 21/14 units										
18–24	35	39	35	36	38	15	19	17	18	18
25–44	31	32	34	33	31	11	13	14	13	14
45–64	21	23	24	25	25	8	8	9	10	11
65+	12	13	13	14	15	3	3	4	5	5
Total	**25**	**27**	**27**	**28**	**27**	**9**	**10**	**10**	**11**	**11**
percentage who drank more than 50/35 units										
18–24	11	14	11	13	11	3	4	3	4	4
25–44	8	8	9	9	7	2	2	2	2	2
45–64	5	5	6	6	6	1	1	1	1	1
65+	2	2	2	3	2	0	0	0	1	0
Total	**6**	**7**	**7**	**7**	**6**	**1**	**2**	**2**	**2**	**2**

UK: (Source: 1992 General Household Survey)

d. UK: In 1992, 28% of people aged 16 and over were cigarette smokers, compared with 30% in 1990; this continues the decline in cigarette smoking that has been monitored by the GHS since the early 1970s. The rate of decline appeared to slow down in the mid-1980s but, since then, it has picked up again, particularly among men. (Source: *Social Trends*, 1995, General Household Survey)

e. UK:

Tobacco consumption per head of population aged 15 and over, 1960–1985

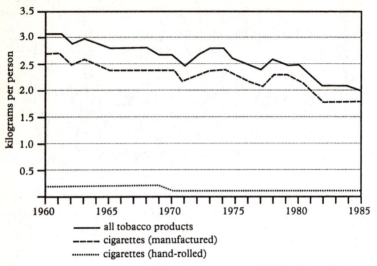

all tobacco products
cigarettes (manufactured)
cigarettes (hand-rolled)

(Source: Graph based on figures taken from *UK Smoking Statistics,* 1988, Nicholas Ward et al, using Tobacco Advisory Council information)

f. UK:

In 1992, a total of 10,784 seizures by police and Customs involved Class A* drugs; 64,654 seizures involved Class B* drugs.

For the police, the rate of Class A drug seizures has increased annually: by 22 per cent in 1990–91 and by 30 per cent in 1991–92.

For Class B drugs – apart from amphetamines – seizure rate increases have slowed: 16 per cent in 1990–91; and 1 per cent in 1991–92.

In 1992, the quantity of heroin seized increased by 10 per cent on 1991, with 550 kg seized; 57 seizures involved quantities of over one kilo, representing almost 90 per cent of the amount seized.

In 1992, there were 2,400 seizures of cocaine, yielding a record 2,248 kg, 59 seizures involved one kilo or more and accounted for over 90 per cent of all cocaine seized.

Seizures of crack cocaine by the police increased by 45 per cent on 1991.

Police seizures of Ecstasy in 1992 increased by 40 per cent although the number of units seized fell by a quarter (from 273,900 to 203,900). Customs seizures, however, though staying at a low number did involve a large quantity (350,000 doses), nearly a 300 per cent increase on 1991.

Seizures of LSD by the police rose 55 per cent on 1991 and the quantity seized was 75 per cent up on 1990's peak figure of 232,600 doses. Customs also seized a record amount – 140,600 doses, a 125 per cent increase on 1990.

Cannabis accounted for 60,000 seizures, some 500 lower that in 1991 – the first recorded fall since 1975. However, quantities seized showed a marked rise.

Seizures of amphetamines have continued to rise steeply and the total provisional quantity seized in 1993 (over 1,000 kg) was over three times more than that seized in 1990.

★ Class A drugs include cocaine, heroin, LSD and morphine. Class B drugs include amphetamines, hashish and marijuana.

(Source: *Tackling Drugs Together*, HMSO Cm 2678, 1994)

5. Marijuana/hashish

a. England: In 1992 cannabis accounted for 60,000 seizures, some 500 lower than in 1991 and the first recorded fall since 1975. However, quantities seized show a marked rise. (Source: *Tackling Drugs Together*, HMSO Cm 2678, 1994)

b. England: 1990–93, 14% of people aged 12–59 had taken cannabis and 24% of 16–29 year olds reported long-term use. (Source: *Tackling Drugs Together*, HMSO Cm 2678, 1994)

7. Alcohol

a. UK: Statistics for 1992 indicate that 24% of boys aged 11–15 and 17% of girls aged 11–15 had an alcoholic drink in the last week. Since 1984 there has been a gradual rise in the number of women exceeding the sensible drinking level. (Source: *Social Trends 25*, 1995)

USA

Use of alcohol in the past month by youths 12–17 years of age, according to age and sex, selected years 1974–91

Age/Sex	1974	1976	1977	1979	1982	1985	1988	1990	1991
12–17	34	32	31	37	27	31	25	25	20
12–13	19	19	13	20	10	11	07	08	07
14–15	32	31	28	36	23	35	23	26	19
16–17	51	47	52	55	45	46	42	38	35
Male	39	36	37	39	27	34	27	25	22
Female	29	29	25	36	27	28	23	24	18

(Source: Health, United States, 1992, Public Health Service)

b. England: The proportion of men drinking more that the sensible maximum fell from 28% in 1990 to 26% in 1992 but among women it rose slightly. (Source: *Social Trends 25*, 1995)

USA: In 1992, more than 7% of adults surveyed met DSM-1V criteria (Diagnostic and Statistical Manual of Mental Disorders, Fourth Edition) for 1-year alcohol abuse, alcohol dependence, or both. Males were almost three times more likely than females to meet the criteria for alcohol abuse and/or dependence. (Source: Prevalence of DSM-1V alcohol abuse and dependence, United States, 1992 [Epidemiologic Bulletin No.35, Alcohol Health and Research World, 1994])

c. UK:

Alcohol, cancer and attributable risk

cancer	attributable to alcohol	number of lives saved: at zero consumption	at half present rate of consumption
larynx	45%	430	94
oesophagus	22%	2699	162
oral/cavity pharynx	45%	267	29
liver	35%	433	62
*breast:	16%	2163	155

There is enough consistency in findings to suggest an association between alcohol and breast cancer; however, there is little evidence yet of a causal link. (Source: alcohol concern information and research bulletin drawing on Duffy, John C: *Alcohol and Illness: the epidemiological viewpoint*, Edinburgh University Press 1992).

Bibliography

Arno Adelaars, *Ecstasy, de opkomst van een bewustzijnsveranderend middel*, Amsterdam 1991.

Adviesburo Drugs Amsterdam en Nederlands Instituut voor Alcohol en Drugs, folder 'XTC, Waarschuwing aan alle XTC-gebruikers', Utrecht maart 1992.

Adviesbureau Drugs August de Loor, Amsterdam, in opdracht van Nederlands Instituut voor Alcohol en Drugs (NIAD), 'Folder XTC', Utrecht 1990.

R. van Amerongen, 'Geschiedenis van de alcoholpreventie' in *Alcoholpreventie, achtergronden, praktijk en beleid* (redactie: J.C. van der Stel, W.R. Buisman), Alphen aan den Rijn/Brussel 1988.

Arta-medewerkers, *Vrije Opvoedkunst*, sociaal-pedagogisch tijdschrift, jaargang 49, nr. 1, januari 1986.

Arta-medewerkers (A. van den Berg et al.), *Rock Bottom, Beyond Drug Addiction*, Stroud (Groot-Brittannië) 1987.

Arta, Jaarverslagen.

Richard Ashley, *Cocaine, Its History, Uses and Effects*, New York 1975.

Arthur Baanders, *'De Hollandse aanpak.' Opvoedingscultuur, drugsgebruik en het Nederlandse overheidsbeleid*, Assen/Maastricht 1989.

J.I. van Baaren, *Zoeklicht op verslaving*, Amsterdam 1968.

Hans-Georg Behr, *Weltmacht Droge, Das Geschäft mit der Sucht*, Wien/Düsseldorf 1980.

P.C. van den Berg, 'Hallucinose en psychose bij cocaïne-gebruik', in *Cocaïne* (red. J. van Limbeek), Bilthoven 1986.

Henri Beunders, 'Verbod schept misdaad: lessen van de drooglegging', in nrc *Handelsblad* 8 september 1989, p. 9.

B. Bieleman, J.J. Bosma, K. Swierstra, 'Cocaïne: van mythe tot probleem' in *Tijdschrift voor alcohol, drugs en andere psychotrope stoffen*, 1990, nr. 1, p. 11–16.

Jochen Bockemühl, *Levensprocessen in de natuur*, Zeist 1982.

Victor Bott, *Antroposofische geneeskunde*, deel i, Zeist 1985. (*Anthroposophical Medicine: An extension of the art of healing*, Harper/Collins, 1985)

E. Buddecke, *Grundriss der Biochemie*, Berlijn 1989.

Walther Bühler, *Meditation als Erkenntnisweg. Bewusstseinserweiterung mit der Droge*, Stuttgart 1972.

Walter Bühler, L.F.C. Mees, Wolfgang Schimpeler, *Rauschgift, Krieg gegen das Ich*, Stuttgart 1980.

William Burroughs, *Junkie*, Amsterdam 1979.

Timothy G. Coffey, 'Beer Street – Gin Lane, Aspekte des Trinkens im 18. Jahrhundert', in *Rausch und Realität, Drogen im Kulturvergleich* (red. Gisela Völger), Keulen 1981.

Sidney Cohen, 'Medizinischer Stand der Marihuana-Forschung' in *Rausch und Realität, Drogen im Kulturvergleich* (red. Gisela Völger), Keulen 1981.

Tom Dardis, *The Thirsty Muse, Alcohol and the American Writer*, New York 1989.

F.M.H.M. Driessen, G. van Dam en B. Olsson, 'De ontwikkeling van het cannabisgebruik in Nederland, enkele Europese landen en de vs sinds 1969' in *Tijdschrift voor alcohol, drugs en andere psychotrope stoffen*, 1989 nr. 1, p. 2–14.

Ron Dunselman, 'Drugs, meesters van schijnoplossing', in *Jonas* 22, 1987, p. 6–7.

Ron Dunselman, 'Marihuana, de droom van het verloren bewustzijn', in *Jonas* 20, 1992, p. 6–9.

Georg Eckert, *Der Isenheimer Altar, seine geistigen Wurzeln und sein spirituell-künstlerischer Gehalt*, Freiburg i. Br. 1980.

J.H. van Epen, *De drugs van de wereld, de wereld van de drugs*, Alphen aan den Rijn/Brussel 1988.

Christian F. Feest, 'Alkohol bei den Indianern Nordamerikas' in *Rausch und Realität, Drogen im Kulturvergleich* (red. Gisela Völger), Keulen 1981.

Wilhelm Fraenger, *Matthias Grünewald*, München 1983.

Nico J. Francken, 'Antroposofische geneeskunst' in *Gezichtspunten, brochure sociale hygiëne*, Zoetermeer 1990.

Eric Fromberg, 'XTC, een nieuwe soft drug', *Tijdschrift voor alcohol, drugs en andere psychotrope stoffen*, 1990, nr. 4, p. 150–158.

Eric Fromberg, *XTC, hard drug of onschuldig genotmiddel?*, Amsterdam/Lisse 1991.

P.J. Geerlings en dr. E.Ch. Wolters (red.), *Verslaving, Een handboek voor arts en hulpverlener*, Utrecht 1980.

J.W. Goethe, *Metamorphose der Pflanzen*, Stuttgart 1977. (*The Metamorphosis of Plants*, Bio-Dynamic Farming and Gardening Association.)

C. Goos, 'Verslaving en verslavingszorg in Europa', in Jack Derks en Marten Hoekstra (red.), *Verslavingszorg, een apart vak*, Utrecht 1991.

R. Goudsmit, 'Haematologische afwijkingen ten gevolge van overmatig alcoholgebruik' in *Tijdschrift voor alcohol, drugs en andere psychotrope stoffen*, 1989, nr. 6, p. 210–212.

Dé Granaat, Theo J. van der Wal, *Jeugd onder drug, een verzameling feiten, meningen en citaten*, Amsterdam 1971.

Gerbert Grohmann, *Die Pflanze, Ein Weg zum Verständnis ihres Wesens*, deel i, Stuttgart 1975, en deel ii, Stuttgart 1981. (*The Plant, Vol. 1: A Guide to Understanding Its Nature*, Bio-Dynamic Farming and Gardening Association, 1989.)

K.F. Gunning, *Kijk op hennep*. ao 1626 (red. C. Meinhardt), Lelystad 1976.

J. van der Haar, H. Jäggi, D. Kretschmann, 'Methadon – "Heilung" mittels Betäubung?', in *Mitteilungsblatt Internationale Vereinigung Anthroposophischer Einrichtungen für Suchttherapie e.v.*, nr. 10, Driebergen 1988.

Bernd Hansen, 'America – Home of the Brave. Vernichtung und Lage der Nordamerikanischen Ureinwohner', in Flensburger Hefte nr. 37: *Indianer*, Flensburg 1992.

G.A.J. Hendriks, G.R.M. Molleman en G.M. Schippers, 'Alcoholgebruik en alcoholproblemen: definities en epidemiologische gegevens' in *Alcohol-preventie, achtergronden, praktijk en beleid* (red. J.C. van der Stel, W.R. Buisman), Alphen aan den Rijn/Brussel 1988.

Helmut Hessenbruch, *Wesen und Sinn des Schmerzens*, Unterlengenhardt/Schweiz 1969.

Karl Heymann, 'Suchtgefahren', in *Bewusstseinserweiterung durch Drogen? Zum Problem der Rauschgiftsucht*, Bazel 1970.

Karl Heymann, 'Das Phänomen des Rausches', in *Bewusstseinserweiterung durch Drogen? Zum Problem der Rauschgiftsucht*, Bazel 1970.

Friedrich Hiebel, 'Die psychedelische Revolution' in *Bewusstseinserweiterung durch Drogen? Zum Problem der Rauschgiftsucht*, Bazel 1970.

M.J. Hoekstra en J. Derks, 'Verslaving, verslavingszorg en verslavingsbeleid in Nederland, een overzicht', in Jack Derks en Marten Hoekstra (red.), *Verslavingszorg, een apart vak*, Utrecht 1991.

Albert Hofmann, verslag van een lezing van Albert Hofmann op 27 februari 1970 in Zürich, in *Bewusstseinserweiterung durch Drogen? Zum Problem der Rauschgiftsucht*, Bazel 1970 (verkorte weergave van de volledige tekst van de voordracht, gepubliceerd in de *Neue Zürcher Zeitung*, nr. 105, 4 maart 1970.

Walter Holtzapfel, *Im Kraftfeld der Organe, Leber, Lunge, Niere, Herz*, Dornach 1990.

J. van Ingen, 'Alcohol en coronairsclerose', in *Tijdschrift voor alcohol, drugs en andere psychotrope stoffen*, 1992, nr. 1, p. 33–35.

J. van Ingen, 'Effecten van marihuana en cocaïne op foetale groei', in *Tijdschrift voor alcohol, drugs en andere psychotrope stoffen*, 1990, nr. 6, p. 231–232.

J. van Ingen, 'Ook darminfarcten door cocaïne', in *Tijdschrift voor alcohol, drugs en andere psychotrope stoffen*, 1990, nr. 6, p. 230–231.

J. van Ingen, 'Spierverval ten gevolge van cocaïne (ofte wel "Cocaine, the continuing story")', in *Tijdschrift voor alcohol, drugs en andere psychotrope stoffen*, 1990, nr. 6, p. 230.

J. Jamin, 'Verboden vruchten, drugpreventie op maat', in Jack Derks, Marten Hoekstra (redactie), *Verslavingszorg, een apart vak*, Utrecht 1991.

Bruce D. Johnson, 'Die englische und amerikanische Opiumpolitik im 19. und 20. Jahrhundert: Konflikte, Unterschiede und Gemeinsamkeiten' in *Rausch und Realität, Drogen im Kulturvergleich* (red. Gisela Völger), Keulen 1981.

Olaf Koob, 'Droge und Suchtentstehung' in *Sucht und Drogen*, Lebenshilfen 5, Stuttgart 1989.

Olaf Koob, *Drogensprechstunde*, Stuttgart 1990.

M. Kooyman, 'De medische aspecten van het drug-gebruik', in *Soft drugs, sociale, medische en juridische aspecten*, samengesteld door Cor Wijbenga, Amsterdam 1970.

D.J. Korf, P. Blanken, A.L.W.M. Nabben en J.P. Sandwijk, 'Ecstasy-gebruik in Nederland' in *Tijdschrift voor alcohol, drugs en andere psychotrope stoffen*, 1990 nr. 5, p. 169–175, Lisse.

Dirk Korf, Peter Blanken, Ton Nabben, *Een nieuwe wonderpil? Verspreiding, effecten en risico's van ecstasygebruik in Amsterdam*, Amsterdam 1991.

Elisabeth Kübler-Ross, *Over de dood en het leven daarna*, Baarn 1985. (*Living with Death and Dying*, Macmillan, 1982.)

Aldo Legnaro, 'Alkoholkonsum und Verhaltenskontrolle – Bedeutungswandlungen zwischen Mittelalter und Neuzeit in Europa', in *Rausch und Realität, Drogen im Kulturvergleich* (red. Gisela Völger), Köln 1981.

Ed Leuw, 'Over gokken en de hernieuwde humanisering van het verslavingsbegrip', *Tijdschrift voor alcohol, drugs en andere psychotrope stoffen*, 1988, nr. 5–6, p. 178–186, Lisse.

Harry Gene Levine, 'Die Entdeckung der Sucht – Wandel der Vorstellungen über Trunkenheit in Nordamerika' in *Rausch und Realität, Drogen im Kulturvergleich* (red. Gisela Völger), Köln 1981.

Harry Gene Levine, 'Mässigkeitsbewegung und Prohibition in den usa', in *Rausch und Realität, Drogen im Kulturvergleich* (red. Gisela Völger, Köln 1981.

B.C.J. Lievegoed, *Ontwikkelingsfasen van het kind*, Zeist 1974.

Bernard Lievegoed, *De levensloop van de mens, Ontwikkeling en ontwikkelingsmogelijkheden in verschillende levensfasen*, Rotterdam 1976.

Bernard Lievegoed, *Mens op de drempel. Mogelijkheden en problemen bij de innerlijke ontwikkeling*, Zeist 1983. (*Man on the Threshold: The Challenge of Inner Development*, Hawthorn Press, 1990.)

J.A. van Limbeek, 'Inleiding', in *Psychiatrie en verslavingszorg*, onder redactie van J. van Limbeek, in samenwerking met W.J. Edelbroek, Bilthoven 1985.

August de Loor, *Het middel Ecstasy bestaat niet. Een onderzoek*, Adviesburo Drugs Amsterdam 1989.

Hans Peter van Manen, *Kaspar Hauser, Zijn leven en zijn plaats in de geschiedenis*, Zeist 1985.

L.F.C. Mees, *De achtergronden van de drugcatastrofe, de mens tussen leiding en verleiding* (oorspronkelijke titel: *Drugs... waarom eigenlijk*), Driebergen-Rijsenburg 1988.

J.D. van der Meulen, 'Drugs en het strafrecht', in *Soft drugs, sociale, medische en juridische aspecten*, samengesteld door Cor Wijbenga, Amsterdam 1970.

Ministerie van Welzijn, Volksgezondheid en Cultuur, *Nota Verslavingsproblematiek*, juni 1992.

Bert Minjon, Roland D.F. Wolters, *Hulpverlening bij verslavingsproblemen, een multimethodische benadering*, Alphen aan den Rijn/Brussel 1988.

Raymond A. Moody jr., *Leven na dit leven. Ervaringen van mensen tijdens hun klinische dood*, Bussum/Naarden 1980. (*Life after Life: The Investigation of a Phenomenon, Survival of Bodily Death*, Walker and Company, 1988.)

Raymond A. Moody, *De tunnel en het licht. Het verschijnsel van de bijna-doodervaring*, Utrecht/Antwerpen 1988. (*The Light Beyond*, Bantam Books.)

Klaus-Dieter Neumann, 'Auf fremden Pfaden, Interview mit Ron Dunselman und Jaap van der Haar über die Wirkungen verschiedener Drogen' in 'Flensburger Hefte' nr. 16, *Kulturvergiftung, Rauschgift, Sucht und Therapie*, Flensburg 1987.

Hans Rudolf Niederhäuser, 'lsd', in *Bewusstseinserweiterung durch Drogen? Zum Problem der Rauschgiftsucht*, Bazel 1970.

Het onkruid en de bloem. Dagboek van een verslaafd meisje, Amsterdam.

Wilhelm Pelikan, *Heilpflanzenkunde* i, ii en iii, Berlijn 1988, 1982 en 1984.

Gert Preiser, 'Wein im Urteil der griechischen Antike', in *Rausch und Realität, Drogen im Kulturvergleich* (red. Gisela Völger), Köln 1981.

F. van Ree, P. Esseveld, *Drugs, de medische en maatschappelijke aspecten*, Utrecht/Antwerpen 1985.

J.M. van Ree, 'Farmacologische werking van cocaïne', in *Cocaïne* (red. J. van Limbeek), Bilthoven 1986.

Udo Renzenbrink, *Anthroposofische voedingsleer*, Zeist 1980.

Gottfried Richter, *Der Isenheimer Altar des Matthias Grünewald*, Stuttgart 1981.

George G. Ritchie, *Terugkeer uit de dood*, Haarlem 1990. (*My Life after Dying*, Hampton Roads Publishing Company, 1991.)

Arman Sahini, *Synthetische drugs. Het nieuwe gevaar*, Rijswijk 1989.

Franziska Sarwey, *Grünewald-Studien, Zur Realsymbolik des Isenheimer Altars*, Stuttgart 1983.

Karl Georg Scheffer, 'Coca in Südamerika' in *Rausch und Realität, Drogen im Kulturvergleich* (red. Gisela Völger), Köln 1981.

Jürgen vom Scheidt, 'Kokain', in *Rausch und Realität, Drogen im Kulturvergleich* (red. Gisela Völger), Köln 1981.

Wolfgang Schmidbauer, Jürgen vom Scheidt, *Handbuch der Rauschdrogen*, Frankfurt am Main 1989.

Martin Schouten, *Marihuana en hasjiesj, een handboek*, Utrecht/Antwerpen 1969.

L. Schrijnemakers, 'Koffie, geprezen en verguisd' in *Arts en auto*, jaargang 55, p. 654, 655.

Richard E. Schultes, Albert Hofmann, *Pflanzen der Götter, Die magischen Kräfte der Rausch- und Giftgewächse*, Bern und Stuttgart 1987.

Bernard Segal, *Drugs and Behavior, Cause, Effects and Treatment*, New York/London 1988.

W.Chr. Simonis, *Genuss aus dem Gift? Herkunft und Wirkung von Kaffee, Tee, Kakao, Tabak, Alkohol und Haschisch*, Stuttgart 1979.

A.G.H. Smals, 'Alcohol en het endocriene systeem', in *Tijdschrift voor alcohol, drugs en andere psychotrope stoffen*, 1989, nr. 4, p. 121–124, Lisse.

Solomon H. Snyder, *Brainstorming, The Science and Politics of Opiate Research*, Cambridge (Massachusetts, usa), Londen (Engeland) 1989.

R. Spieksma, *Alcoholisme, diagnostiek, pathofysiologie en enkele richtlijnen voor behandeling*, Maassluis 1989.

Alfred Springer, *Kokain, Mythos und Realität, Eine kritisch dokumentierte Anthologie*, Wien-München 1989.

Rudolf Steiner, *Alte und Neue Einweihungsmethoden* (ga 210), Dornach 1967.

Rudolf Steiner, *Beroep en karma* (ga 172), Zeist 1991.

Rudolf Steiner, *Het christelijk opstandingsmysterie en de voorchristelijke mysterië* (ga 8), Zeist 1985.

Rudolf Steiner, *De drempel van de geestelijke wereld. Aforistische beschouwingen* (ga 17), Zeist 1975.

Rudolf Steiner, *Dromen, hallucinaties, visioenen. Openbaringen van het onbewuste*, Amsterdam 1990; voordracht 21 maart 1918.

Rudolf Steiner, *De filosofie der vrijheid. Grondtrekken van een moderne wereldbeschouwing. Resultaat van observaties op zielsgebied volgens natuurwetenschappelijke methode* (ga 4), Cothen 1989.

Rudolf Steiner, 'Das Geheimnis des Erforschens anderer Welten durch die Metamorphose des Bewusstseins', voordracht 14 augustus 1924 in *Das Iniaten-Bewusstsein* (ga 243), Dornach 1983.

Rudolf Steiner, *Geisteswissenschaft und Medizin* (ga 312), Dornach 1985.

Rudolf Steiner, *Geisteswissenschaftliche Menschenkunde* (ga 107), Dornach 1988.

Rudolf Steiner, *Gemeinsamheit über uns, Christus in uns* (uit ga 159/160), Dornach 1989.

Rudolf Steiner, *Gezondheid en ziekte* (ga 348), Zeist 1984.

Rudolf Steiner, *Lachen en huilen* (uit ga 59), Amsterdam 1987.

Rudolf Steiner, *Het leven van mens en aarde* (uit ga 349), Zeist 1983.

Rudolf Steiner, *Natuur en mens, geesteswetenschappelijk beschouwd* (ga 352), Zeist 1978; voordracht 11 januari 1912.

Rudolf Steiner, *Nervositeit. Een levensprobleem*, Zeist 1987.

Rudolf Steiner, *De opvoeding van het kind in het licht van de antroposofie*, Zeist 1986.

Rudolf Steiner, *Theosofie. Inleiding tot bovenzintuigelijke kennis van de wereld en van de bestemming van de mens* (ga 9), Zeist 1985.

Rudolf Steiner, *Voordrachten over het evangelie volgens Johannes* (ga 103), Zeist 1984.

Rudolf Steiner, *Een weg naar zelfkennis in acht meditaties* (ga 16), Zeist 1979.

Rudolf Steiner, *De weg tot inzicht in hogere werelden* (wv-d1; ga 10), Bilthoven 1991.

Rudolf Steiner, *De wetenschap van de geheimen der ziel* (ga 13), Zeist 1989.

Rudolf Steiner, *Zeitgeschichtliche Betrachtungen. Das Karma der Unwahrhaftigkeit – Erster Teil* (ga 173), Dornach 1978.

Rudolf Steiner, *Zeitgeschichtliche Betrachtungen. Das Karma der Unwahrhaftigkeit – Zweiter Teil* (ga 174), Dornach 1983.

Rudolf Steiner, Ita Wegman, *Grondslagen voor een verruiming van de geneeskunde volgens geesteswetenschappelijke inzichten* (ga 27), Zeist 1981.

J.C. van der Stel, 'Alcoholpreventie en de ontwikkeling van gezondheidsbeleid', in *Alcoholpreventie, achtergronden, praktijk en beleid* (red. J.C. van der Stel, W.R. Buisman), Alphen aan den Rijn/Brussel 1988.

Michael Stolleis, 'Von dem grewlichen Laster der Trunckenheit, Trinkverbote im 16. und 17. Jahrhundert', in *Rausch und Realität, Drogen im Kulturvergleich* (red. Gisela Völger), Köln 1981.

René Stoute, *Op de rug van vuile zwanen*, Amsterdam 1982.

Andreas Suchantke, 'Orientierungsversuche im Labyrinth der Drogen', in *Bewusstseinserweiterung durch Drogen? Zum Problem der Rauschgiftsucht*, Bazel 1970.

K. Swierstra, 'Heroïneverslaving: levenslang of gaat het vanzelf over?' in *Tijdschrift voor alcohol, drugs en andere psychotrope stoffen*, 1987 nr. 3, p. 78–92, Leidschendam

J. Tholen, S. Siero en G.J. Kok, 'Gevolgen van alcoholgebruik tijdens de zwangerschap' in *Tijdschrift voor alcohol, drugs en andere psychotrope stoffen*, 1988 nr. 2, p. 41–49, Lisse.

Bram Tjaden, 'Psychose – een onvoorbereide grensovergang' in *Jonas 23*, 5 juli 1985.

Rudolf Treichler, *Die Entwicklung der Seele im Lebenslauf. Stufen, Störungen und Erkrankungen des Seelenlebens*, Stuttgart 1981. (*Soulways: The Developing Soul-Life Phases, Thresholds and Biography*, Hawthorn Press, 1990.)

Rudolf Treichler, *Seelische Entwicklung und Sucht*, Stuttgart 1988.

Alfred Usteri, *Pflanzen-Wesen*, Dornach 1989.

Vakgroep Verslavingszorg, *Cocaïne, de parel osnder de zwijnen*, Arta-Zeist 1990.

Arie Visser, *Het vangen van de draak, een boosaardig verhaal*, Amsterdam 1983.

Felicitas Vogt, *Drogen, Sekten, New Age. Bewusstseinserweiterung um jeden Preis?*, Dornach 1992.

Irmgard Vogt, 'Alkoholkonsum, Industrialisierung und Klassenkonflikte', in *Rausch und Realität, Drogen im Kulturvergleich* (red. Gisela Völger), Köln 1981.

J.A. Walburg, 'Verslavingshulpverlening in het fin de siècle' in Jack Derks en Marten Hoekstra (red.), *Verslavingszorg, een apart vak*, Utrecht 1991.

Wolfgang Weirauch, 'Der mürbe Becher, Interview mit Dr. Heinz Harmut Vogel', in Flensburger Hefte nr. 17: *Kulturvergiftung. Alkohol*, Flensburg 1987.

Wolfgang Weirauch, 'Küsse die der Teufel gibt, Interview mit Dr. Olaf Titze', in Flensburger Hefte nr. 17: *Kulturvergiftung. Alkohol,* Flensburg 1987.

G.A.M. Widdershoven en R.H.J. ter Meulen, 'De drinker of de drank? Het alcoholisme-concept in de 19e en 20e eeuw' in *Tijdschrift voor alcohol, drugs en andere psychotrope stoffen,* 1989, nr. 3, p. 105–112, Lisse.

Otto Wolff/Walter Bühler, 'Weltproblem Alkohol', in *Sucht und Drogen,* Lebenshilfen 5, Stuttgart, 1989.

F.W. Zeylmans van Emmichoven, *De menselijke ziel. Inleiding tot de kennis van het wezen, de werkzaamheid en de ontwikkeling van de ziel,* Zeist 1974.

W.M. de Zwart, *Alcohol, tabak en drugs in cijfers,* Utrecht 1989.

Coen van Zwol, 'Markt voor nederwiet is vrijwel verzadigd', in nrc *Handelsblad,* 17 februari 1993, p. 2.

The St Brendan Group of Great Britain

A small group of people (The St Brendan Group) have it in their sights to found a residential community with drug misusers in Britain. This group is inspired by Arta – the therapeutic community in The Netherlands where the author, Ron Dunselman, works.

Further information can be obtained from:

Frank O'Hare/Kenny Thomson
71 Bridgeburn Drive
Woodiesburn by Chryston
Glasgow G69 0AT

Other books from Hawthorn Press

Parenting for a healthy future

Dotty T Coplen

'Nobody ever told me about children,' said one bemused parent. Here is a commonsense approach to the challenging art of parenting; an offer of genuine support and guidance to encourage parents to believe in themselves and their children. Dottie Coplen helps parents gain a deeper understanding of parenting children from both a practical and holistic, spiritual perspective. The book posits sensible suggestions and invaluable insights into ways of bypassing the inevitable hurdles of parenting without compromising the enjoyment of the process.

216 x 138mm; limp bound
ISBN 1 869 890 53 1

Voyage through childhood into the adult world: a guide to child development

Eva A Frommer

Human beings have a long infancy during which they are dependent upon others for the means of life and growth – such a book on child development is therefore vital. Many of Frommer's ideas in this book derive from her professional observations as a child psychiatrist and include her personal distillations of Rudolf Steiner's teachings. A deep concern for the uniqueness of each individual child permeates this book, while offering practical solutions to the challenges of raising a child at each stage of his or her development.

216 x 138mm; 140pp approx; paperback;
colour and black & white photographs
ISBN 1 869 890 59 0

Raising a son: parents and the making of a healthy man

Don Elium and Jeanne Elium

Many parents feel frustrated and confused by the behaviour of their sons and are in need of some practical guidance during the various stages of their son's development into manhood. *Raising a Son* offers just that advice on firm but fair discipline that will encourage the awakening of your son's healthy soul. The book will prove useful not only to both single and married parents, but to all men and women who deal with children.

Between form and freedom: a practical guide to the teenage years

Betty Staley

Betty Staley offers a wealth of insights about teenagers, providing a compassionate, intelligent and intuitive look into the minds of children and adolescents. She explores the nature of adolescence and looks at teenagers' needs in relation to family, friends, schools, love and the arts. Issues concerning stress, depression, drug and alcohol abuse and eating disorders are included.

210 x 135mm; 288pp; sewn limp bound; illustrations
ISBN 1 869 890 08 6

The twelve senses

Albert Soesman. Translated by Jakob Cornelis.

The senses nourish our experience and act as windows on the world. But our stimulation may undermine healthy sense experiences. The author provides a lively look at the senses, not merely the normal five senses, but twelve: touch, life, self-movement, balance, smell, taste, vision, temperature, hearing, language, the conceptual and the ego senses. The imaginative approach provides an accessible study guide for teachers, doctors, therapists, counsellors, psychologists and scientists.

210 x 135 mm; 176pp; sewn limp bound
ISBN 1 869 890 22 1

Soulways: the developing soul: life phases, thresholds and biography

Rudolf Treichler. Translated by Anna Meuss

Soulways offers insights into personal growth through the phases and turning points of human life. A profound picture of child and adult development is given, including the developmental needs, potentials and questions of each stage. Drawing on his work as a psychiatrist, Treichler also explores the developmental disorders of soul life – addictions, neuroses, hysteria, anorexia and schizophrenia.

210 x 135mm; 320pp; sewn limp bound
ISBN 1 869 890 13 2

Tools for transformation: a personal study

Adam Curle

This exploration of mediation, development and education draws on case studies from disparate cultural and geographical sources, reminding us of our participative relationship with the fabric of life. Specific issues include approaches to violence, negotiation, the nature of democracy, consensus management, community development, non-violence and learning for life.

210 x135mm; 224pp; sewn limp bound
ISBN 1 869 890 21 3

If you have difficulties ordering from a bookshop you can order direct from

Hawthorn Press,
Hawthorn House,
1 Lansdown Lane,
Lansdown,
Stroud,
Glos.
United Kingdom,
GL5 1BJ

Telephone 01453 757040
Fax 01453 751138